FEEDING
THE FRASERS

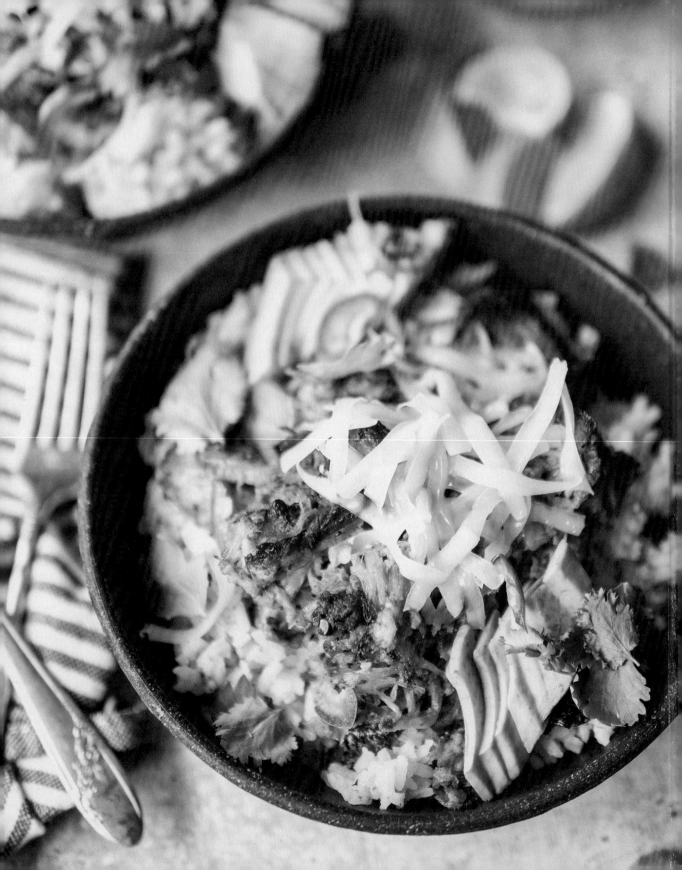

FEEDING
THE FRASERS

FAMILY FAVORITE RECIPES
MADE TO FEED THE FIVE-TIME
CROSSFIT GAMES CHAMPION,
MAT FRASER

SAMMY MONIZ

ST. MARTIN'S GRIFFIN

NEW YORK

First published in the United States by St. Martin's Griffin, an imprint of St. Martin's Publishing Group

FEEDING THE FRASERS. Copyright © 2021 by Sammy Moniz. All rights reserved. Printed in the United States of America. For information, address St. Martin's Publishing Group, 120 Broadway, New York, NY 10271.

www.stmartins.com

Photographs and recipes by Sammy Moniz

The Library of Congress Cataloging-in-Publication Data is available upon request.

ISBN 978-1-250-77602-0 (trade paperback)
ISBN 978-1-250-77603-7 (ebook)

Our books may be purchased in bulk for promotional, educational, or business use. Please contact your local bookseller or the Macmillan Corporate and Premium Sales Department at 1-800-221-7945, extension 5442, or by email at MacmillanSpecialMarkets@macmillan.com.

First Edition: 2022

10 9 8 7 6 5 4 3 2 1

To the *Feeding the Frasers* well-fed family, I cannot thank you enough for your never-ending support. Thank you for showing up each day, re-creating recipes for your family and sharing them through Instagram, emails, messages, and comments. I feel the support and love watching your inspiration in the kitchen spread.

To my family and friends, thank you for your support and for always being there to take home the leftovers!

To my sweetheart, Mat. Thank you for the daily encouragement to follow my passion. Thank you for being an incredible example of **hard work** and for your constant support. You are the inspiration behind every meal. I appreciate *you,* each taste test, and all the feedback you've given to this project over the years. This one is dedicated to you!

CONTENTS

SIDES, SALADS & SANDWICHES

SNACKS & SWEETS

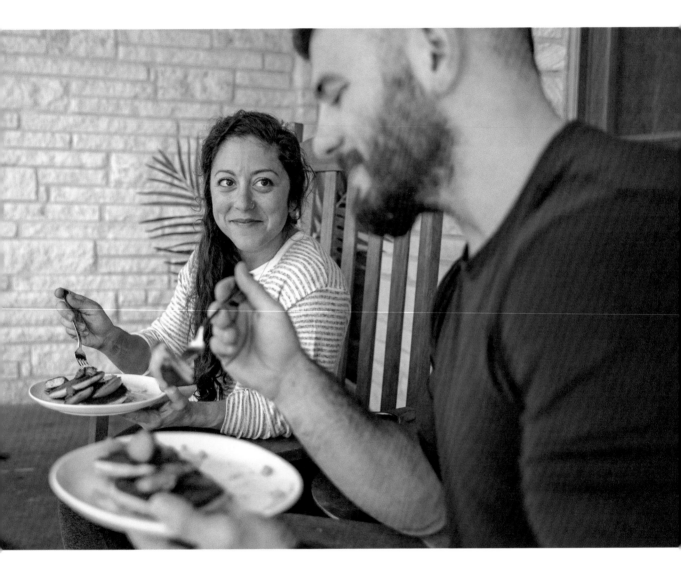

INTRODUCTION

I didn't grow up cooking alongside my grandmother or mom. It wasn't a part of my family culture. Cooking, as I remember it, was a chore. As one of five kids in a small house with seven people and one shared bathroom, mealtime was not elaborate. It was whatever could hit the table at a reasonable hour to feed the family amid the bustle of sports practices and homework. There was a simple rotation of meals that could feed our large family on a budget—spaghetti and meat sauce, casserole, shepherd's pie, and tacos. I know my mom didn't enjoy the process, but who could blame her? Cooking for a small army with big opinions on what they like or dislike is a daunting task, even for those who enjoy time in the kitchen. Looking back, I genuinely don't remember if the meals were good or bad. What sticks with me is the effort my parents made to bring us together at the end of the day for a meal. *That* is from where my curiosity around cooking stems. Food is so tightly connected to our memories. Whether it's the memory of Mom's American Chop Suey (see page 94 for recipe) or the memories of shared time around the dinner table, I want to foster these memories for my family and friends.

Cooking not only feeds my family, it feeds my own personal creativity. I learned how to cook through cooking. Want to master the perfect bagel? Bust out the flour and make a few batches of bagels! Soon, the task of boiling and baking bagels won't seem as daunting. The recipe begins to feel more and more familiar. The results, better and better with each batch. The recipes you'll find here are the ones that helped me learn. Some are simple, and others require a little more time. Take it at your own pace, enjoy the process, and use this book as a tool to learn, grow, and bring people together around food. I cannot wait for you to experiment and get creative with the recipes I share in this book. I look forward to seeing you gathering around the table, with your people, brought together by your dedicated efforts and *dayummmm* good food.

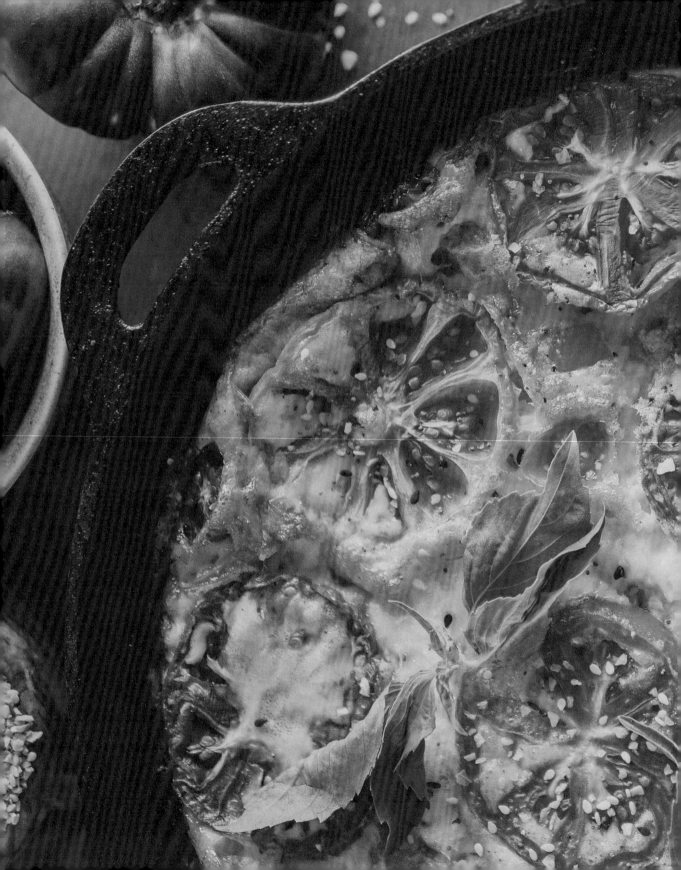

BREAKFAST: SAVORY

THE SEVEN-MINUTE EGG

SERVES: 4
PREP TIME: 5 MINUTES
COOK TIME: 7 MINUTES

8 eggs

IN OUR house, the soft-boiled egg is king. It's the ultimate showstopper addition to any meal. The Well-Fed Fraser is always impressed by perfectly oozing yolks. If only he knew how easy they were! The sweet spot for us is 7 minutes, but we've tried everything from 6–10 minutes. We found 7 minutes is just enough time to fully cook the whites and set the edge of the yolk, while also giving you a soft and runny yolk to mix into your dish. Whether it be the topper to a warm bowl of ramen, mixed into a summer salad, or a toast topper for breakfast, these soft-boiled eggs will be the perfect addition to any meal.

Bring a large pot of water to a rolling boil. Using a slotted spoon, lower each egg into the water, careful not to crack the shells as they touch the bottom of the pot. Set the timer for 7 minutes.

While the eggs boil, fill a large mixing bowl with ice water. Set the bowl near the stove. When the 7 minutes is complete, remove each egg from the pot and place it into the bowl of ice water. Let the eggs cool in the ice bath for 2 minutes. Remove the shells, slice, and enjoy with your favorite dish.

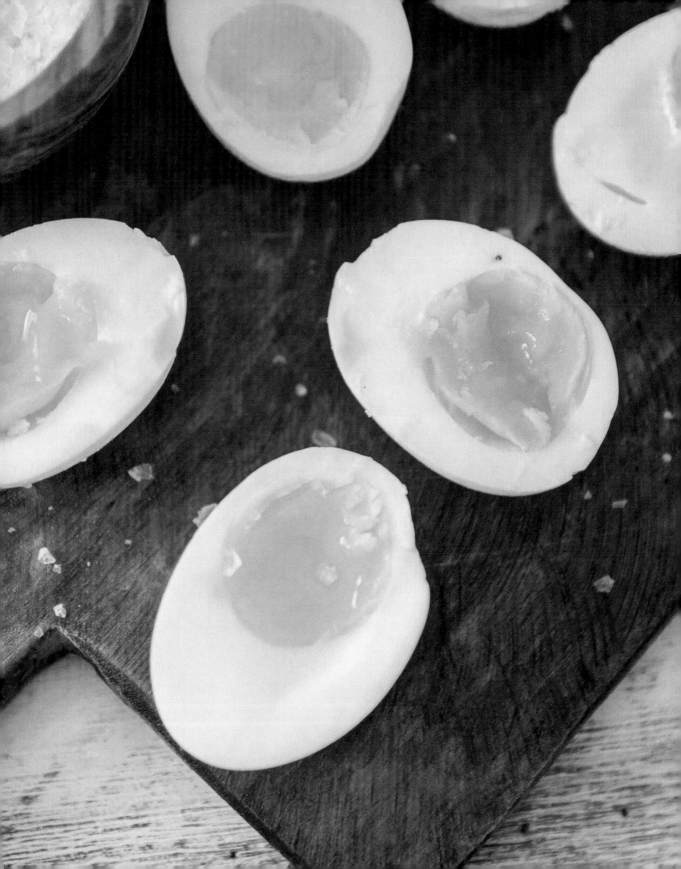

HERBY EGG PLATE

SERVES: 4
PREP TIME: 20 MINUTES
COOK TIME: 7 MINUTES

4 ounces spring mix salad

¼ cup fresh herbs (parsley, cilantro, basil), roughly chopped

1–2 tablespoons olive oil

Flaky salt

1 pint cherry heirloom tomatoes, halved

8 ounces cheddar cheese, cubed small

8 Seven-Minute Eggs (see page 2 for recipe), peeled and quartered

4 tablespoons basil pesto, homemade or store bought

EVERY SUMMER after Mat completes his CrossFit competition season, we spend time in Canada at our cabin on the lake. We stay in a tiny little town with nothing to do other than sip coffee on the dock and listen to the loons. In this one-traffic-light town, there's a hip coffee shop in an old, small church. I look forward to our daily trips during our stay for a sweet treat and espresso or a sit-down meal. The most surprising menu item to me is, for lack of a better explanation, a breakfast salad. I was sold! I like to re-create a version of that breakfast salad and re-live the end of summer at the lake at least once a month at home. It's amazing how food is so closely tied to our memories. I think about that often when preparing meals for friends and family. Each time I serve a meal, I'm hoping to imprint memories of warmth, joy, and good times.

In a large mixing bowl, toss the spring mix and herbs. Drizzle with olive oil and add a pinch of flaky salt. In another small bowl, toss the tomatoes with a pinch or two of flaky salt. Add the tomatoes to the large mixing bowl along with the cheddar cheese. Toss to combine.

Assemble each plate by evenly distributing the herby mixed greens. Top each salad with two Seven-Minute Eggs, drizzle each plate with a little basil pesto over the eggs, and serve.

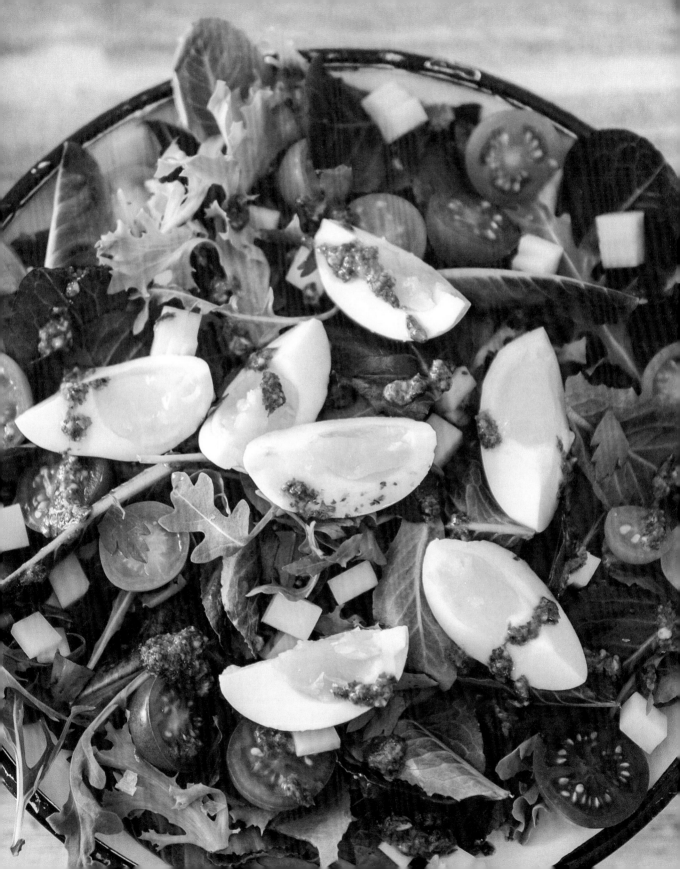

BAKED CHIPOTLE BREAKFAST TACOS

SERVES: 4
PREP TIME: 10 MINUTES
COOK TIME: 35–40 MINUTES

8 slices thick-cut bacon

1 tablespoon salted butter

8 eggs

1 teaspoon salt

2 ounces sharp cheddar cheese, diced or shredded

8 corn tortillas, warmed

1 tablespoon olive oil

1 cup greek yogurt

⅓ cup cilantro, finely chopped

1 tablespoon chipotles in adobo with sauce, finely chopped

1 ripe avocado, quartered for serving

TACOS ARE amazingly versatile. You can have them any time of day. You can tuck a variety of ingredients into a flour or corn tortilla and have a new and exciting bite each time.

Preheat the oven to 350°F/177°C. Line a baking sheet with aluminum foil, lay strips of bacon on the sheet, leaving space between each. Bake in the oven for 15–20 minutes.

While the bacon bakes, heat the salted butter in a large, nonstick skillet over low heat. Whisk the eggs and salt. Cook the eggs for 5–7 minutes, pushing around the skillet until eggs are just about set. Add the cheese to the eggs, mix until incorporated and melted, about 2 minutes. Remove the eggs from the heat.

Remove the bacon from the oven, place it on a paper towel–lined plate, set aside. Increase the oven temperature to 425°F/220°C.

Microwave the corn tortillas for 30 seconds, up to 1 minute, until pliable. With your hands, rub each tortilla with olive oil and place on a baking sheet. Fill each tortilla with 1 slice of bacon and eggs evenly distributed throughout. Fold the tortillas, bake in the oven for 8 minutes. Flip and return to the oven for an additional 5 minutes until crispy and browned.

Meanwhile, in a small bowl, mix the greek yogurt, cilantro, and chipotles in adobo. Set aside for serving.

Serve tacos with a dollop of chipotle yogurt, avocado slices, and any other desired toppings (e.g., sliced jalapeños, cilantro, pickled onions).

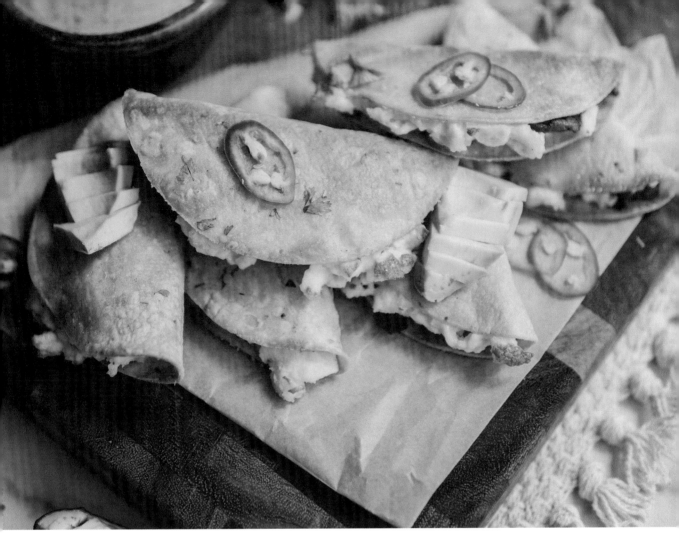

PRO TIP

Microwave the tortillas before stuffing. It's a seemingly simple step to skip, but beware the results are vastly different. If you want cracked and limp tacos, by all means, don't warm the tortillas, but I can tell you from experience, it's not the way to go.

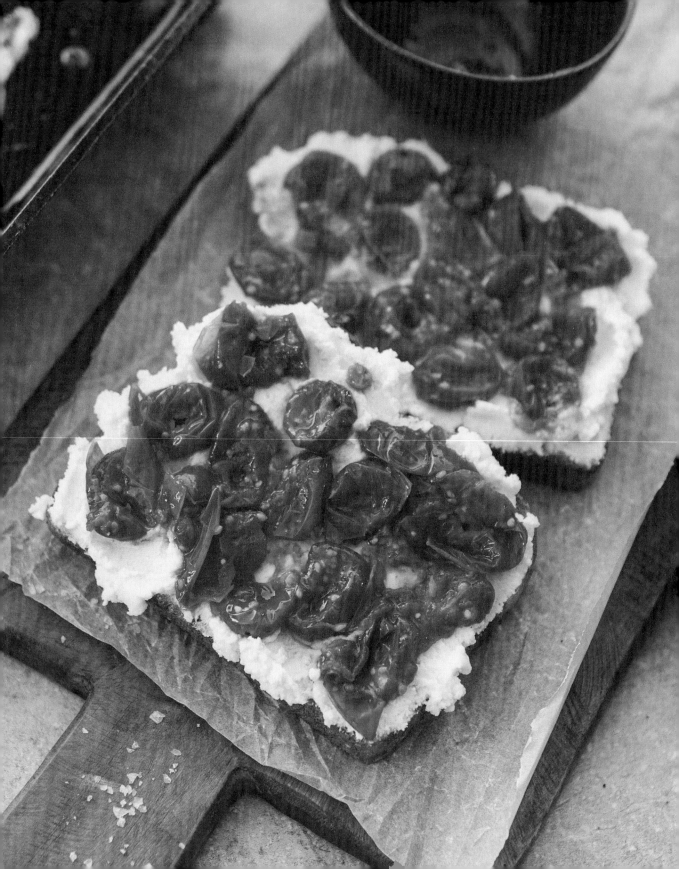

SMOKED TOMATOES, WHIPPED RICOTTA & FRIED EGGS

SERVES: 4
PREP TIME: 10 MINUTES
COOK TIME: 5 MINUTES

16 ounces ricotta cheese

2 tablespoons olive oil

8 eggs

8 slices bread, toasted

Smoked Tomatoes (see page 148 for recipe)

I LOVE toast for breakfast. It's a blank canvas on which to paint the day. This is a simple recipe packed with a ton of flavor. Feel free to add some fresh herbs like basil or even a drizzle of basil pesto to the top of the egg for added freshness and to make the smoked tomatoes pop.

For the whipped ricotta, simply place the ricotta into the bowl of a food processor and whip for 1–2 minutes, until smooth.

Pour 2 tablespoons of olive oil in a large, nonstick skillet over medium heat. When the oil shimmers, crack the eggs into the pan and cook for 3–4 minutes. This amount of time will deliver set whites and a runny yolk; cook longer for your desired doneness.

To assemble, evenly distribute the whipped ricotta to the toasted bread. Top with the warmed smoked tomatoes and a fried egg.

WHIPPED FETA & EGG TOASTIE

SERVES: 4
PREP TIME: 15 MINUTES
COOK TIME: 7–10 MINUTES

8 large eggs

4 Persian cucumbers, sliced thin and quartered

Kosher salt

8 ounces whipped feta (see page 185 for recipe, great use of leftovers!)

1–2 tablespoons fresh dill, plus more for garnish

8 slices sourdough bread, toasted

THIS IS a true leftovers creation. One evening, I'd made a big batch of whipped feta for entertaining friends and the next morning decided to spread it over toast. This is tzatziki-meets-morning toast. The fresh, crisp cucumbers and dill with salty whipped feta are just begging for an oozy yolk to bring it all together.

Bring a large pot of water to a rolling boil. Using a slotted spoon, lower each egg into the water, careful not to crack the shells as they touch the bottom of the pot. Set the timer for 7 minutes. Fill a large mixing bowl with ice water. Set the bowl near the stove. After 7 minutes, remove each egg from the pot and place into the bowl of ice water. Let the eggs cool in the ice bath for 2 minutes.

While the eggs cool, bring your other ingredients together.

In a medium bowl, toss the thinly sliced cucumbers with a pinch of kosher salt. Let the cucumbers sit for 5 minutes. To the bowl, add the whipped feta and fresh dill, set aside.

Once the eggs have rested, remove them from the water bath, crack, and remove the shells.

To assemble your toastie, evenly distribute the cucumber feta spread onto each slice of toasted bread. To each slice, add an egg, quartered into smaller pieces. Top with additional fresh dill—1 serving is 2 slices of smeared toast.

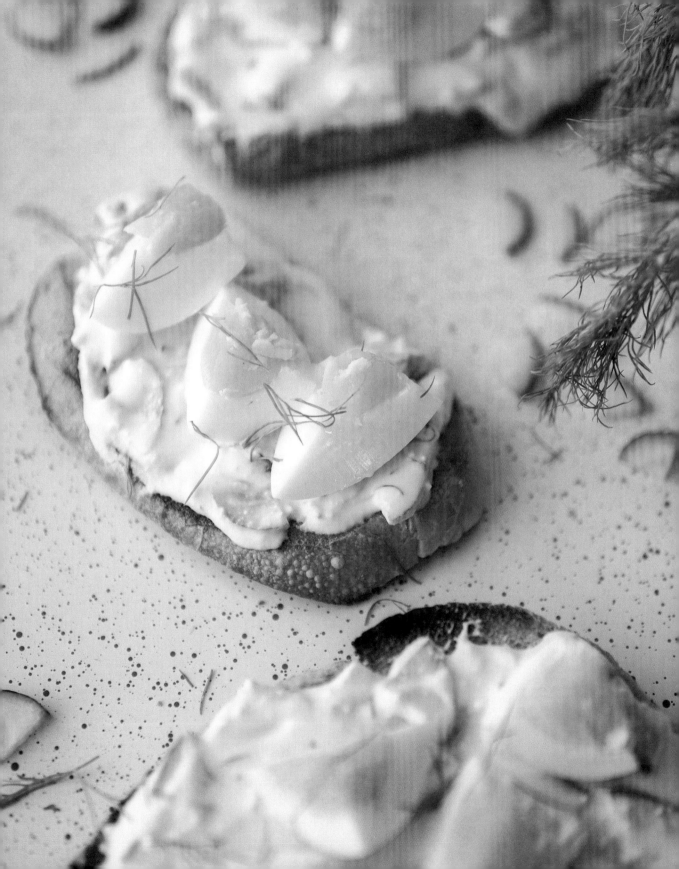

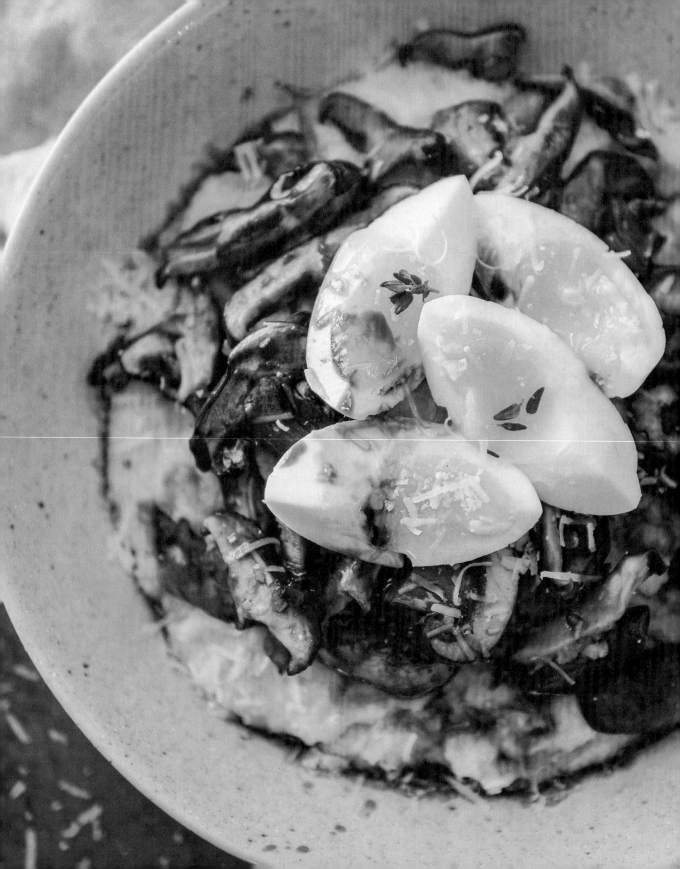

ROASTED MUSHROOM POLENTA BOWL

SERVES: 4

PREP TIME: 10 MINUTES

COOK TIME: 1 HOUR

2 pints cremini mushrooms, sliced

2 pints shiitake mushrooms, sliced

1 shallot, minced

1 garlic clove, minced

5¼ cups chicken broth, divided

2 tablespoons olive oil

2–3 sprigs fresh thyme

1 cup polenta

½ cup freshly grated Parmesan cheese, plus more for serving

8 Seven-Minute Eggs (see page 2 for instructions)

MAT IS a big fan of mushrooms, and it's often his request for added veggies to any breakfast scramble dish. Since I'm always trying to keep mealtimes interesting, this hearty and wholesome meal is perfect for cozy mornings. It warms you from the inside and keeps you well fed until your next meal.

Preheat the oven to 325°F/165°C. While the oven preheats, add mushrooms, shallot, garlic, ¼ cup of broth, olive oil, and thyme to a 9x13 glass baking dish. Mix well. Cover the dish with aluminum foil, place in the preheated oven for 30 minutes.

After 30 minutes, remove the aluminum foil from the dish and pour the excess liquid from the baking dish into a small saucepan and set aside. Return the mushrooms to the oven, uncovered, and increase the oven temperature to 450°F/230°C. Roast for an additional 20–30 minutes.

While the mushrooms roast, prepare the polenta. To a medium saucepan, add the remaining 5 cups of broth and bring to a boil. Reduce the heat to medium. While whisking constantly, slowly add polenta and bring it to a simmer. Reduce the heat to low, cover, and cook for 30–35 minutes. Whisk the polenta every 10–15 minutes until thick and smooth. In the last 2 minutes, add the freshly grated Parmesan and stir to combine.

While the polenta is cooking and the mushrooms finish roasting, prepare the soft-boiled eggs and bring the mushroom broth to a simmer.

To assemble, scoop a generous serving of polenta into a bowl and top with the roasted mushrooms, top with quartered soft-boiled eggs, a drizzle of the mushroom broth and a sprinkle of Parmesan cheese.

ROASTED POTATO & FENNEL RIB HASH

SERVES: 4

PREP TIME: 10 MINUTES

COOK TIME: 45 MINUTES

1 pound baby gold potatoes, quartered

2 tablespoons olive oil, divided

Salt and pepper to taste

1 cup fresh broccoli, minced

6–8 ounces Fennel Ribs (See page 83 for recipe, great for leftovers!), chopped

8 eggs

¼ cup freshly grated Parmesan for serving

I LOVE hash dishes because they are a great way to tuck leftovers from dinner into a dish, top with an egg, and *poof!* you've got breakfast. Whenever I make ribs, you can bet the leftovers will be served up just like this. If there even are leftovers, of course!

Heat a large cast-iron skillet over medium heat. In a large bowl, toss the quartered potatoes with 1 tablespoon of olive oil, salt, and pepper until fully coated. Add the potatoes to the warmed skillet, cover, and cook for 30 minutes, tossing every 5–7 minutes. Add the minced broccoli and toss to combine. Lastly, add the chopped ribs to the potatoes and cook uncovered until warmed through and the potatoes are soft and browned, about 5–7 minutes.

While the potatoes are cooking, heat a large, nonstick skillet over medium heat with the remaining tablespoon of olive oil. Working in batches, crack the eggs into the pan and cook until the whites are set and the yolks are runny, about 3–5 minutes or until desired doneness.

Serve the potato rib hash topped with 1–2 fried eggs and an additional sprinkle of Parmesan cheese.

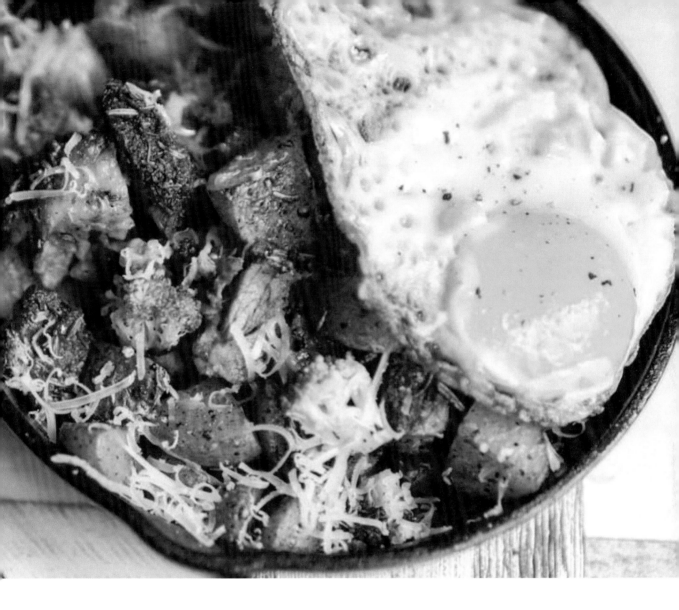

SPICY SHAKSHUKA

SERVES: 4
PREP TIME: 10 MINUTES
COOK TIME: 40 MINUTES

1 pound pork breakfast sausage

1 shallot, minced

1 tablespoon olive oil

1 zucchini, quartered and diced

Kosher salt to taste

½ cup bell pepper, diced

1 (28-ounce) can crushed tomatoes

2 (15-ounce) cans fire-roasted tomatoes

2 teaspoons smoked paprika

1 teaspoon cumin

¼ cup Piri Piri Sauce (see page 60 for recipe)

8 eggs

4 ounces feta cheese, for garnish

Fresh parsley or cilantro, for garnish

IF I sit down at a brunch spot and shakshuka is on the menu, I'm likely to order it. I love the warm stewed tomatoes, hidden veggies, and the oozy yolk to dip a toasted english muffin or crusty bread into. I like spice any time of day, and this recipe features a sneaky leftover. In our house, if I make something for dinner, you're likely to find remnants of it in breakfast the next day. It's how I learned to be creative with food, limit waste, and repurpose ingredients. If you've made the Piri Piri Chicken Wings and have a jar of Piri Piri in the fridge, add a scoop of that flavorful sauce to this dish for an extra kick to get the morning jump-started. If you're looking to make this vegetarian-friendly, swap the breakfast sausage for cooked lentils.

Heat a well-seasoned, large, cast-iron skillet over medium heat. Add the breakfast sausage. Break up the sausage from its packaged form, spread it out, and leave it to cook for 5 minutes. Resist the urge to push it around; this will help a crust form. Once the sausage is almost cooked through and little pink remains, begin to break it up into tiny pieces. Add the minced shallot and cook until no pink remains.

Push the sausage to one side of the skillet, then add the olive oil, zucchini, and a pinch of salt. Cook the zucchini for 3–5 minutes until lightly browned. Add the bell pepper, crushed tomatoes, and fire-roasted tomatoes. Stir to incorporate. Add the smoked paprika, cumin, and Piri Piri Sauce. Reduce the heat to low and simmer for 10 minutes, or until the tomatoes have slightly thickened. Taste and adjust salt as needed.

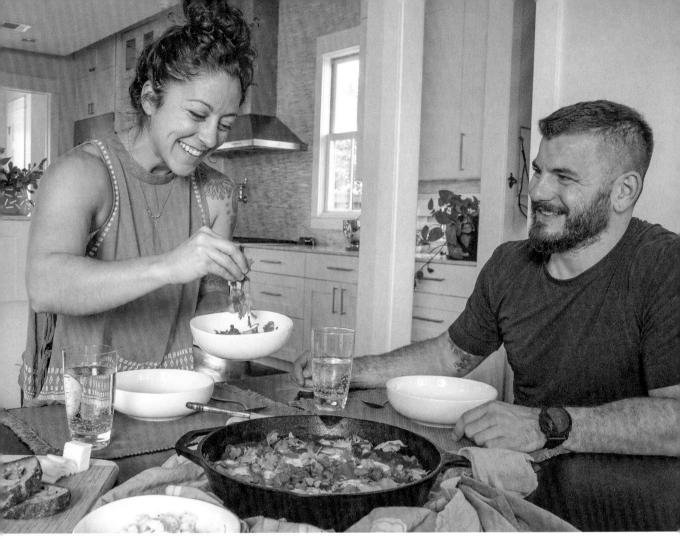

Using a spoon, make a well in the sauce and crack an egg into the well. Repeat with all eight eggs. Cover the pan and cook on low for 5–7 minutes or until the eggs are set.

Garnish the shakshuka with crumbled feta and fresh herbs. Serve with a side of grilled bread or Fennel-Roasted Sweet Potatoes (page 147).

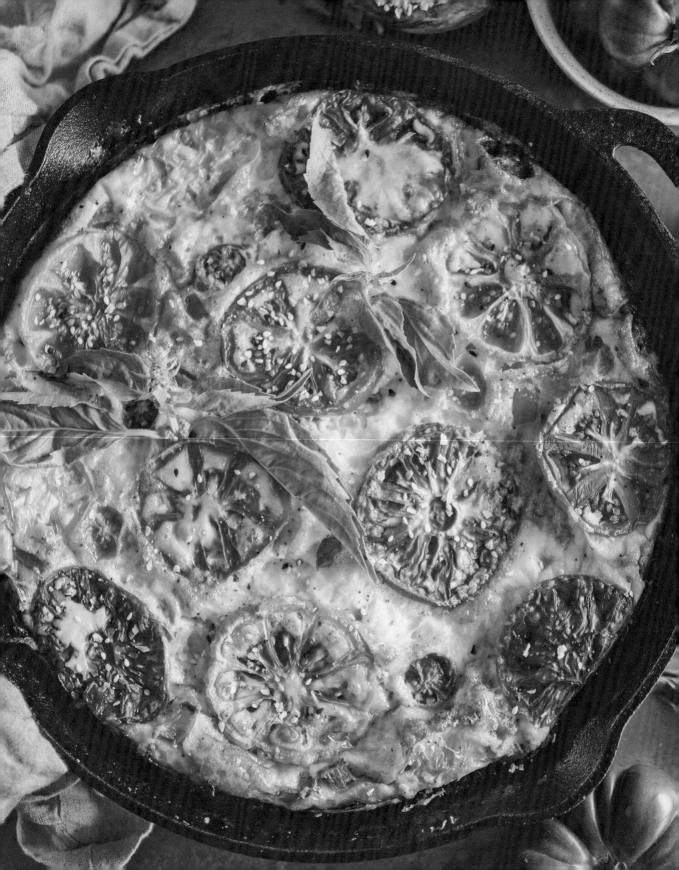

HEIRLOOM & CHEDDAR SUMMER FRITTATA

SERVES: 6–8
PREP TIME: 5 MINUTES
COOK TIME: 60 MINUTES

2 tablespoons olive oil

1 pound ground turkey

1 tablespoon basil pesto

Salt and pepper to taste

16 eggs, whisked

⅓ cup heavy cream

1 cup bell pepper, chopped

6 ounces sharp cheddar cheese, cubed

1–2 large heirloom tomatoes, thickly sliced

1 tablespoon Everything Bagel seasoning

2 tablespoons fresh basil, for serving

FRITTATAS ARE great for entertaining, perfect for weekly meal prep, and ideal for sneaking some extra vegetables into a meal. It's a one-pan wonder! If we've got company coming over or a busy week ahead, I know I can quickly toss together a delicious meal and be as creative as my fridge and pantry ingredients allow. This Heirloom and Cheddar Summer Frittata features our favorite summer ingredient, the heirloom tomato, and pops of sharp cheddar cheese.

Preheat the oven to 375°F/190°C.

Heat the olive oil in a large skillet over medium-high heat. When the oil shimmers, add the ground turkey to the pan. Break it up from its packaged puck to spread it out, but then resist the urge to push it around; this will help create a crust and texture in the turkey. Cook until little pink remains, and then begin to break it up into small pieces, about 7 minutes. Add the basil pesto, cook for an additional minute. Taste, season with salt and pepper, and set aside.

In a large bowl, whisk the eggs and heavy cream with a pinch or two of salt and pepper.

Spray a 9x13 baking dish with cooking spray. Add the cooked ground turkey, bell peppers, whisked eggs, and cubes of cheddar to the pan. Stir to fully incorporate. Add the slices of tomato to the top of the egg mixture. Sprinkle each tomato with a little salt and pepper.

Bake for 45–50 minutes or until the eggs in the center no longer jiggle. Remove the pan from the oven and allow to cool and set for 5 minutes for slicing. Top with fresh basil for serving.

BREAKFAST: SAVORY

ONION BAGEL & STREET CORN CREAM CHEESE

SERVES: 8
PREP TIME: 2½ HOURS
COOK TIME: 40 MINUTES

2 tablespoons salted butter

3 cups sweet onion, finely diced

2 tablespoons white wine

300 ml warm water

4½ teaspoons granulated sugar

2 teaspoons active dry yeast

500 grams bread flour

1½ teaspoons salt

1 tablespoon olive oil

1 egg, whisked

NOTHING SAYS labor of love like homemade bagels. The recipe and process is surprisingly easy, but they require a little elbow grease and a patient cook. Truth be told, much of this recipe is simply passive waiting time while the dough rises. Grab a book, play a card game with your sweetheart, or use the time to cook up the next meal. I promise you'll thank your patient self when you're eating fresh boiled and baked bagels.

Heat a large skillet over medium heat, add the butter. Once the butter has melted, add the diced onions and reduce heat to low. Cook, stirring often, for 12–15 minutes. Add white wine to the pan and continue to cook for an additional 3–5 minutes until all the alcohol has burned off and the onions are a dark golden. Place the caramelized onions in a bowl and cool to room temperature.

Warm the water to 110°F/45°C. Pour 100 ml of the warm water into the bowl of a stand mixer. Add the granulated sugar and stir until it has dissolved. Sprinkle the dry active yeast onto the top of the water and set aside for 5–10 minutes to bloom. The dry active yeast will bubble and foam.

In a large mixing bowl, measure flour and salt, stir to combine, and set aside.

Once the yeast has bloomed, add ½ of the flour and with the dough hook attached begin to mix on low. Mix for 1 minute. Add the remaining flour, and pour 90 ml of water and ½ of the cooled caramelized onions into the mixer as it works. Allow the dry bits of flour to fully soak up the water before adding more. (NOTE: You might not use the remaining 90 ml of water depending on the humidity and altitude of your kitchen.) Knead

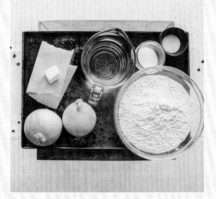
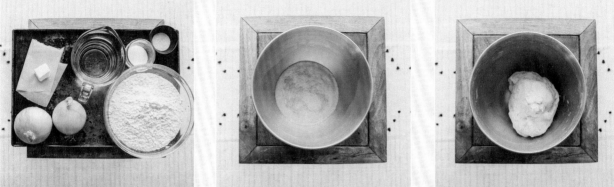
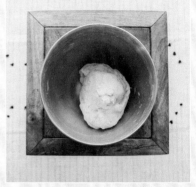

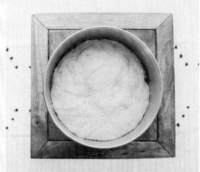
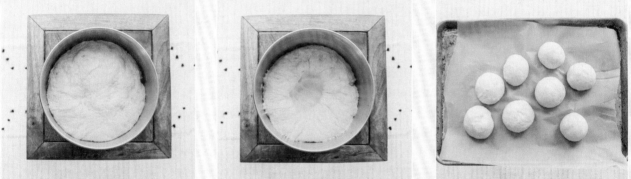
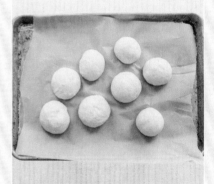

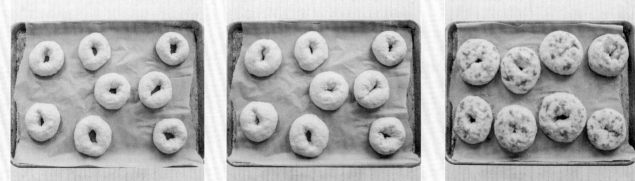
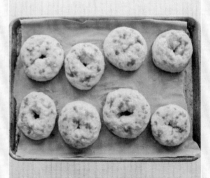

the dough for 10 minutes until a smooth ball forms and pulls away from the sides of the bowl.

Remove the dough from the bowl. Pour the olive oil into the bowl and use a paper towel to fully coat the sides. Return the dough to the oiled bowl, cover with a damp kitchen towel, and place in a warm spot in the kitchen for at least an hour or until the dough has doubled in size.

After the first rise, punch the dough down to deflate it. Cover it again and let it rise another 30 minutes.

Turn the dough out onto a lightly floured surface. Knead for 2–3 minutes until smooth. Using a sharp knife, cut the dough into 8 sections. Smooth each section into a ball by pushing it into the counter with the palm of your hand while making a circular motion. Push your thumb through the center of the ball and work your hands around the dough to form your bagel shape. Place the dough onto a parchment-lined baking sheet. Cover the tray of shaped bagels with a damp kitchen towel to rise for 20 minutes.

When ready to bake, preheat the oven to 425°F/220°C. Bring a large pot of water to a rolling boil. Whisk one egg in a small bowl, and set aside.

Boil each bagel for 1 minute on each side. Place the boiled bagels on a sheet of parchment paper. Brush each boiled bagel with the egg wash, then evenly distribute the remaining caramelized onions to the tops of each bagel. Move bagels to a dry parchment-lined baking sheet. Bake at 425°F/220°C for 18–20 minutes or until golden.

STREET CORN-WHIPPED CREAM CHEESE

SERVES: 8
PREP TIME: 15 MINUTES
COOK TIME: 20 MINUTES

1 ear of corn, husked

1 teaspoon olive oil

Salt and pepper to taste

¼ cup crumbled cotija cheese

Zest of 1 lime

½ teaspoon chili powder

1 green onion, sliced

8 ounces cream cheese, room temperature

Preheat the grill to 450–500°F/230–260°C. Place the corn on a baking sheet, drizzle with olive oil, and season with salt and pepper. Grill 5-7 minutes per side until cooked and charred.

Remove the corn from the grill and cool for 5-10 minutes. Using a sharp knife, remove the charred kernels from the cob and place in a small bowl. To that bowl, add cotija cheese, lime zest, chili powder, and green onion. Mix until well incorporated.

In a medium bowl, whip the room temperature cream cheese using a hand mixer until fluffy, about 2 minutes. Gently fold the corn into the whipped cream cheese using a silicone spatula. Serve Street Corn-Whipped Cream Cheese spread over an onion bagel.

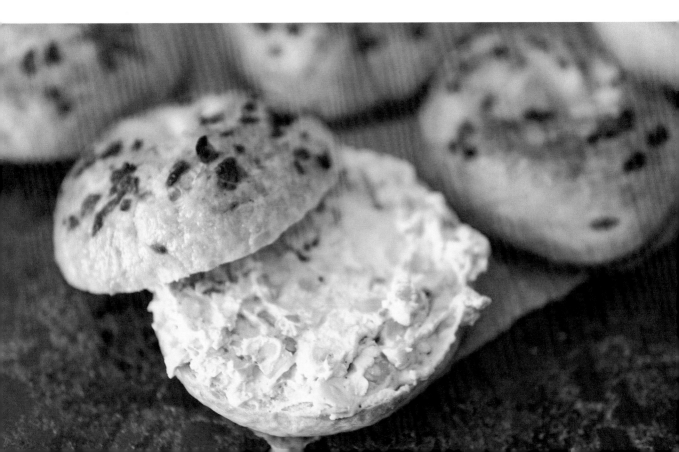

CORN CAKE FRITTER, JALAPEÑO HONEY BUTTER, AND SWEET & SPICY BACON

FRITTERS AND BACON

8 slices thick-cut bacon

1 tablespoon honey

1 teaspoon cayenne pepper, divided

½ teaspoon cracked black pepper

1 cup masa harina

½ cup all-purpose flour

1 tablespoon granulated sugar

2 teaspoons baking powder

1 teaspoon kosher salt

2 cups fresh corn kernels

½ medium jalapeño pepper, seeded
and minced (optional)

2 tablespoons green onion, minced

½ cup heavy cream

2 large eggs

½ cup plus 2–4 tablespoons olive oil

Soft scrambled eggs
for serving

SAVORY AND sweet delicate hot cakes for breakfast? Yes, please! Packed with corn kernels, minced jalapeño, and minced green onion, the cake-to-filling ratio is just enough to keep the ingredients together. Try to resist slathering each bite with the Jalapeño Honey Butter, I dare you!

Preheat the oven to 350°F/177°C. On an aluminum foil–lined baking sheet, lay the strips of bacon down. Drizzle the bacon with honey, add ½ teaspoon cayenne and black pepper, and spread with your hands. Bake for 20–25 minutes or until desired doneness. Remove from the oven, lay on a paper towel–lined plate, cover with aluminum foil to keep warm, and set aside for serving.

In a medium bowl, mix masa harina, all-purpose flour, granulated sugar, baking powder, salt, and the remaining ½ teaspoon of cayenne pepper. Toss the corn kernels, minced jalapeño (if using), and green onion with the dry ingredients, using your hands to fully coat. In a separate bowl, whisk the heavy cream, eggs, and ½ cup of olive oil. Pour the wet ingredients into the dry and stir to combine.

Heat a large cast-iron skillet over medium heat, add the remaining 2 tablespoons of olive oil. When the oil shimmers, scoop the corn cake batter into your hand using a ¼ measuring cup, press to flatten between your palms. Cook 2–3 minutes on each side until golden brown. Move to a paper towel–lined plate and cover with aluminum foil to keep warm while you cook the remaining batter.

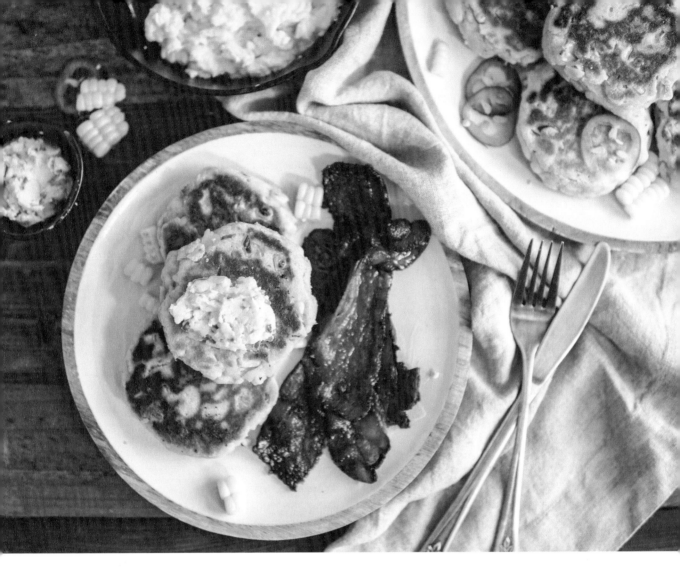

JALAPEÑO HONEY BUTTER

4 tablespoons salted butter, room temperature

1 tablespoon honey

2 teaspoons jalapeño, finely diced

For the Jalapeño Honey Butter, using a hand mixer, or some elbow grease, whip the softened butter, honey, and diced jalapeños. Set aside for serving.

Stack 3 pancakes high, dollop a serving of jalapeño honey butter. Serve with sweet-and-spicy bacon and a side of soft scrambled eggs.

SAUSAGE BUTTERMILK BISCUITS

SERVES: 6
PREP TIME: 35 MINUTES
COOK TIME: 30 MINUTES

8 ounces breakfast sausage

3 cups all-purpose flour

1 tablespoon baking powder

¾ teaspoon baking soda

2 teaspoons salt

¾ teaspoon sugar

1 cup salted butter, grated
(chilled in the freezer)

1 cup buttermilk, cold

1 egg plus 1 tablespoon
heavy cream, whisked

6 tablespoons maple syrup,
for brushing

THESE ARE big and beautiful, just the way a biscuit should be! I want flaky biscuits that topple over because they get so much height in the oven. These are a treat in our house. You wouldn't find them on the menu every week, but it's a recipe that gets your hands involved, and that's why it's in this book. It's a recipe that brings the learning to life. When we can get in there and get dirty with our hands, the end result is that much sweeter. Or that much butterier.

Heat a cast-iron skillet over medium heat, spread the breakfast sausage out evenly over the surface of the pan. Resist the urge to push it around for at least 3–5 minutes to allow a crust to form. When little pink remains, break it up into small pieces. Once the sausage is fully cooked through, remove the sausage from the pan onto a paper towel–lined plate to cool for 15 minutes. Move the sausage to a fresh paper towel–lined plate and place the plate in the refrigerator/freezer to chill completely before making your biscuit dough.

Place flour, baking powder, baking soda, salt, and sugar in a large bowl, and mix with your hands to combine. Add the grated butter, toss to fully coat in flour and distribute. Add the cooked and chilled sausage, tossing to fully coat and distribute.

Add the buttermilk and work the dough with your hands until the buttermilk is fully incorporated and the dough is no longer dry. The dough should be slightly shaggy but hold together before transferring to a flour-dusted surface.

Working with your hands, mold the dough into a rough rectangle. Using a sharp knife, cut the rectangle in half lengthwise. Cut each length in half, leaving you with

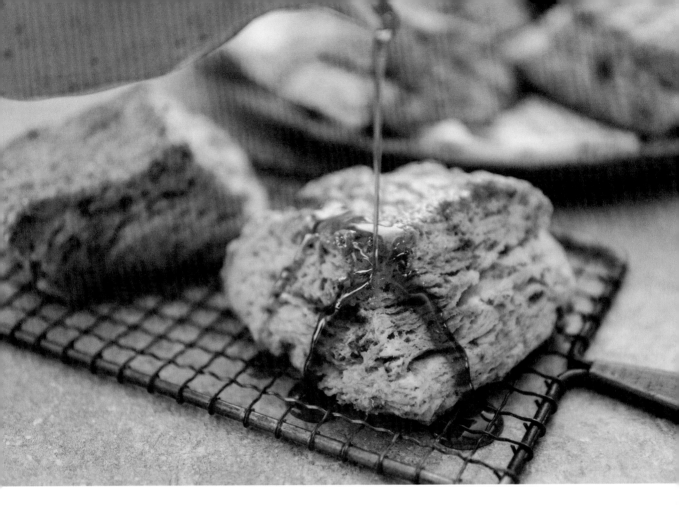

four segments. Pile the segments on top of each other, creating a tall stack of dough. Lightly dust your rolling pin and beat the stack down. Roll out into another rectangle. Repeat this step again.

For the final time, roll out the dough into a rectangle; the height should be about 1–1½ inches thick. Cut the dough in a 3×2-inch grid to create 6 square biscuits.

Place the cut biscuits on a parchment-lined ¼ baking sheet. Brush the tops of each biscuit with the egg and cream mixture. Place the biscuits in the freezer for 20 minutes while the oven preheats.

Preheat the oven to 400°F/200°C. Bake the biscuits for 20–25 minutes until golden brown.

When the biscuits have about 2 minutes remaining, remove the tray from the oven, quickly brush the tops of the biscuits with maple syrup, and return to the oven.

Remove the biscuits from the oven and cool on a wire rack for 2 minutes. Serve each biscuit with an additional drizzle of maple syrup to taste.

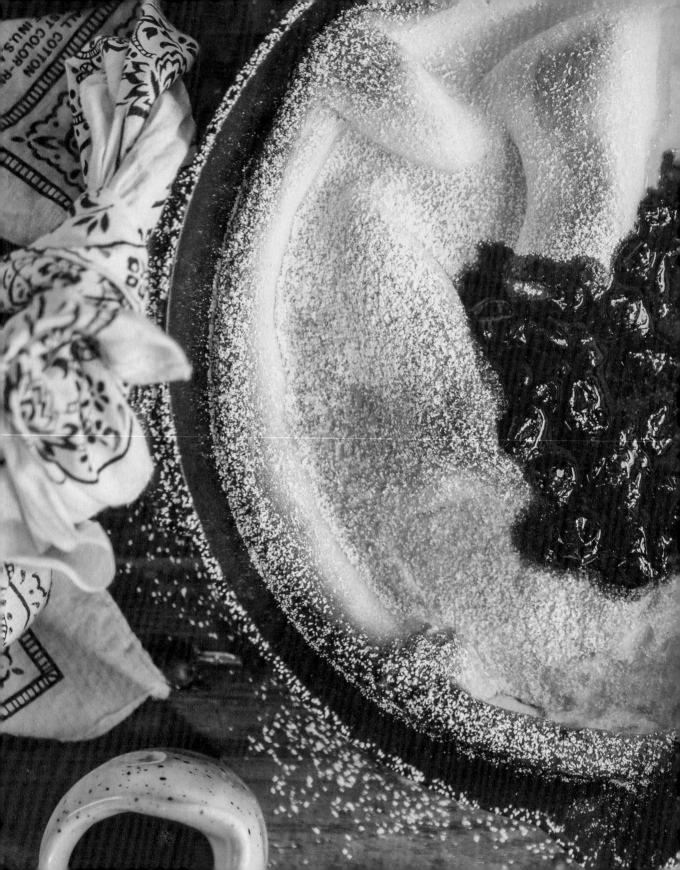

BREAKFAST: SWEET

BAKED & GRILLED SWEET POTATO WITH NUT BUTTER, GRANOLA & HONEY

SERVES: 4
PREP TIME: 5 MINUTES
COOK TIME: 10 MINUTES

4 sweet potatoes, baked

1 tablespoon olive oil

4 tablespoons nut butter of choice

½ cup Hickory-Smoked Pecan Granola (see page 52 for recipe)

4 tablespoons honey

Pinch flaky salt

THIS RECIPE came to be with leftovers from dinner the night before. I baked extra sweet potatoes, because if I'm going to turn the oven/grill on and bake something for 40–60 minutes, I might as well double down and have leftovers. We also happened to be out of bread, and all I really wanted was some toast. One thing led to another and I had charred sweet potatoes and a mountain of flavor and texture. It was a happy little accident, and I'm more than happy to be sharing it with you!

Preheat the grill to 450–500°F/230–260°C.

Cut each sweet potato in half lengthwise, drizzle the olive oil onto the cut-side of the sweet potato. When the grill is to temperature, place the sweet potatoes cut-side down for 7–10 minutes until charred and warmed through.

Remove the sweet potatoes from the grill, slather each with a tablespoon of nut butter, a handful of granola, and a drizzle of honey. Top with an additional pinch of flaky salt to taste.

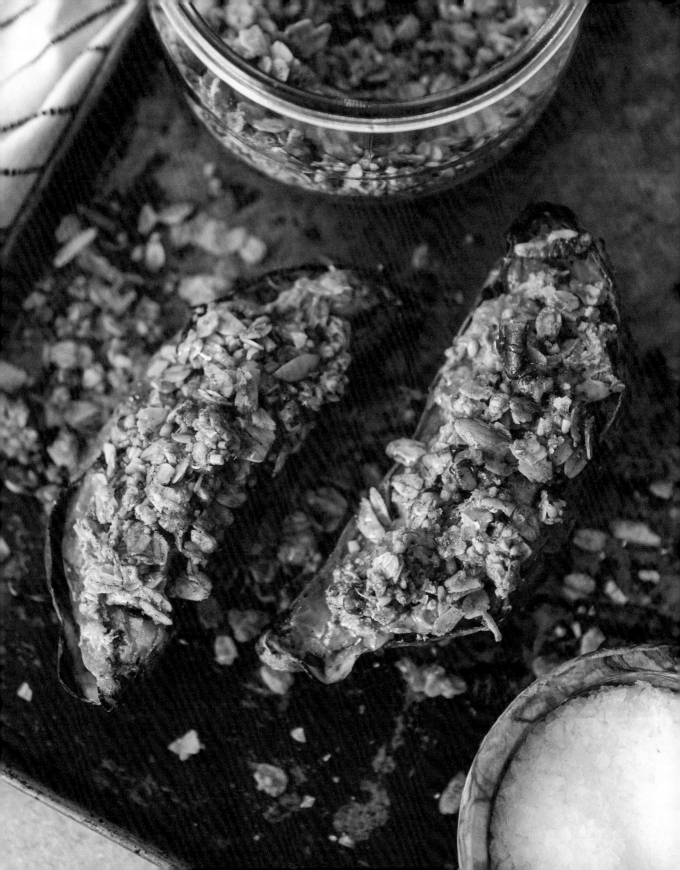

GINGER-SWEET POTATO PANCAKES

YIELDS: 12 PANCAKES
PREP TIME: 10 MINUTES
COOK TIME: 25–30 MINUTES

2 cups all-purpose flour

2 cups sweet potatoes, mashed

2 eggs

2 cups ginger beer (I suggest Reed's zero sugar)

2 tablespoons salted butter, divided

2 cups blueberries

2 tablespoons maple syrup, plus more for serving

1 cup vanilla Greek yogurt for serving

THE KEY to this recipe is cooking on low heat. The ginger beer not only provides flavor and a touch of sweetness but gives lift to the pancake from the carbonation. Feel free to swap for a plain sparkling beverage and customize your flavor with spices like cinnamon and nutmeg instead of the ginger from the ginger beer. A friend made us a version of these pancakes, and I was blown away by the toppings. I'll never go back to serving a stack of pancakes with *just* maple syrup.

Using a stand mixer on low, mix the flour, sweet potato, and eggs. Pour 1 cup of ginger beer into the batter and mix on low with the stand mixer. Pour the remaining 1 cup of ginger beer into the batter and use a silicone spatula to fold the batter until smooth.

Preheat a large, nonstick skillet over low heat.

For each batch of pancakes, melt 1 teaspoon of butter in the warmed pan to prevent sticking. Using a ¼ measuring cup, scoop 2–3 pancakes into the skillet. Cook for 2–3 minutes or until the bottom is browned. Flip the pancakes and cook for an additional 2–3 minutes. Repeat with the remaining batter.

While the pancakes are cooking, heat a small skillet or saucepan over medium heat. Add the blueberries with 2 tablespoons of maple syrup and heat for 5–7 minutes until bursting and juicy. Remove from the heat and set aside.

When ready to serve, place 3–4 pancakes on each plate. Top the stack with the bursting blueberries, a cool dollop of greek yogurt, and a drizzle of maple syrup.

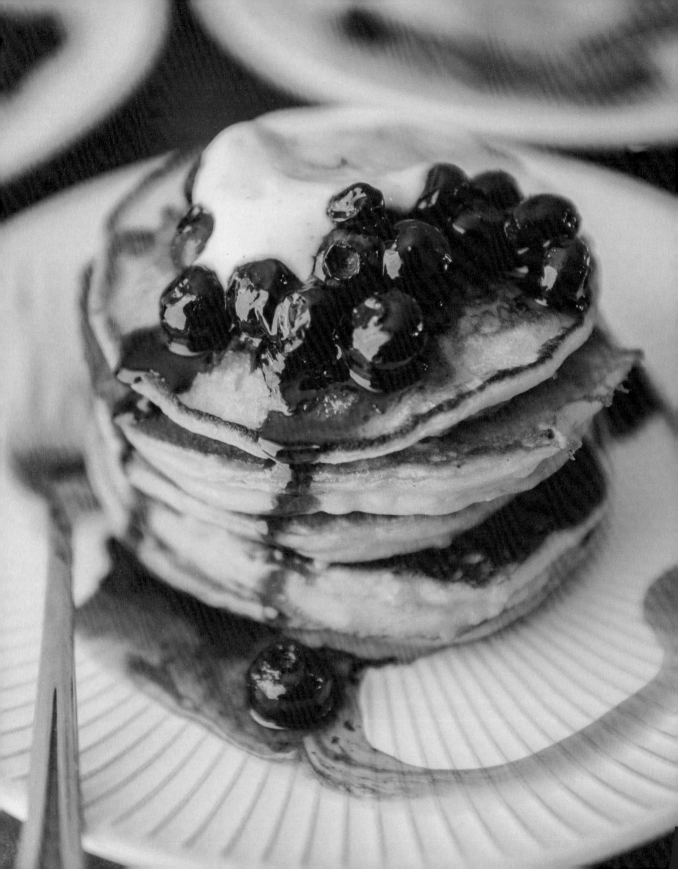

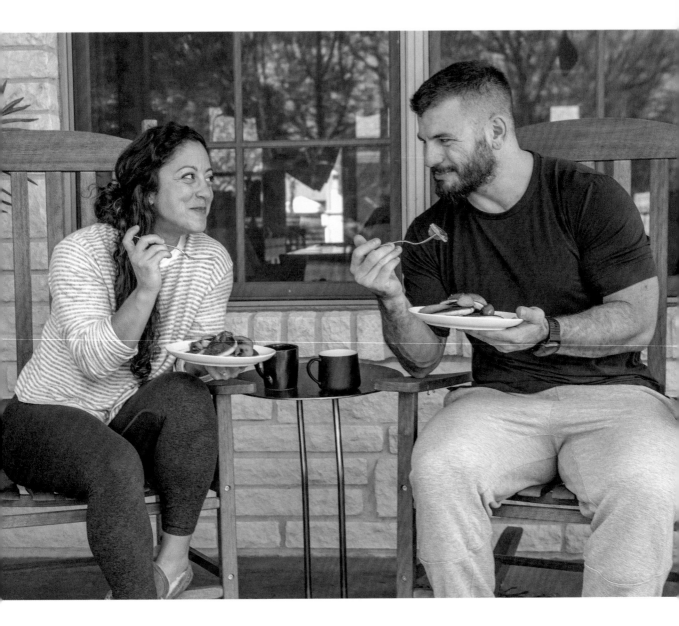

RICOTTA-PEACH PANCAKES

YIELDS: *12 PANCAKES*
PREP TIME: *10 MINUTES*
COOK TIME: *15 MINUTES*

2 eggs, separated

8 ounces ricotta

¾ cup buttermilk

1 teaspoon vanilla extract

1 cup all-purpose flour

½ teaspoon baking soda

¼ teaspoon salt

3 tablespoons salted butter, divided

2 peaches (or nectarines), sliced

2 tablespoons brown sugar

2 tablespoons maple syrup, plus more for serving

THE FIRST time I made ricotta pancakes for the Well-Fed Fraser, my sweetheart asked, "Why are ricotta pancakes not the standard for pancakes?" What an amazing question! They are truly the perfect pancake and so, in our house, this is the standard.

Using a hand mixer, beat egg whites on high speed until stiff peaks form, about 5 minutes. Set aside.

In a large bowl, whisk the egg yolks, ricotta cheese, buttermilk, and vanilla extract until combined. In a separate bowl, whisk the flour, baking soda, and salt. Mix dry ingredients into the large bowl of wet ingredients. In two batches, gently fold the whipped egg whites into the batter. Do not overmix.

Heat a large skillet over medium heat. Melt 1 teaspoon of butter for each batch. Scoop out the batter using a ¼ measuring cup. Cook until the pancakes bubble on top and then flip, about 2–3 minutes per side.

While the pancakes are cooking, prepare the peach topping. Heat a large skillet with 2 tablespoons of butter over medium heat. Once the butter is melted and fragrant, cook sliced peaches for 2–3 minutes on each side until soft. Add the brown sugar and maple syrup, reduce heat to low, and cook an additional 2 minutes.

Serve a stack of pancakes with a scoop of peaches and an additional drizzle of maple syrup as desired.

TRIPLE-BERRY PANCAKE BAKE

1 batch Ricotta Pancakes
(see page 35 for recipe)

3 eggs

¾ cup whole milk

¼ cup heavy cream

2 tablespoons maple syrup,
plus more for serving

1 teaspoon vanilla extract,
divided

Cooking spray

½ cup fresh strawberries,
quartered

½ cup fresh blueberries

½ cup fresh blackberries

¼ cup brown sugar

1 tablespoon lemon zest

¼ cup all-purpose flour

¼ cup quick-cook oats

¼ teaspoon cinnamon

3 tablespoons salted butter,
room temperature

Maple syrup, for serving

OVERNIGHT BAKES remind me of the holidays and big family brunch gatherings. When my family gets together for a holiday celebration or brunch, everyone is in charge of a staple breakfast item. There was always some form of overnight bake. Soft and sweet with a perfectly set custard drizzled with maple syrup. Slice into this Triple-Berry Pancake Bake for a delicious bite and a stunning display of layer on top of layer of pancakes and berries.

To start, see the recipe on page 35 for Ricotta Pancakes, make 2 batches.

In a medium bowl, whisk the eggs, whole milk, heavy cream, maple syrup, and 1 teaspoon of vanilla extract.

Spray a 9x13 baking dish with cooking spray. Cut the pancakes in half and stand the pancakes up against each other cut-side down. Pour the egg mixture on top. Cover and chill at least 2 hours and up to overnight.

When ready to bake, preheat the oven to 350°F/177°C.

In a small bowl, toss the strawberries, blueberries, blackberries, brown sugar, lemon zest, and 1 teaspoon of vanilla until combined.

In a separate small bowl, combine the flour, oats, cinnamon, and butter, working with your hands to fully incorporate into a crumb mixture.

Add the berries, working them in between the pancake halves. Top with the oat crumb. Bake until golden and center is set, about 50–60 minutes. If the crumb topping browns before the bake is set, cover loosely with aluminum foil and continue to bake until done.

Allow the bake to cool for 15 minutes before slicing. Serve with a drizzle of maple syrup.

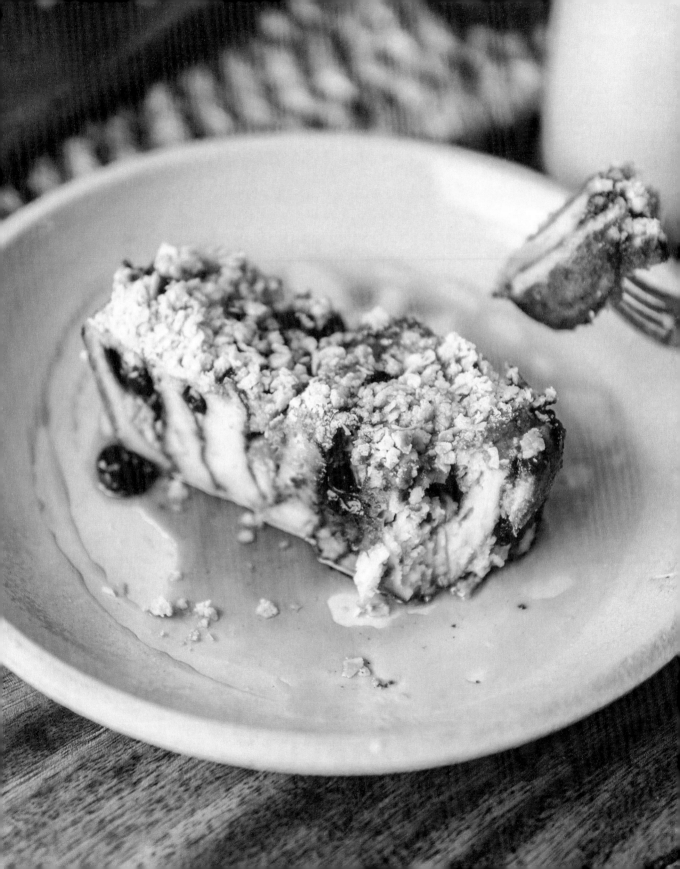

DUTCH BABY WITH LEMON-THYME BLUEBERRIES

SERVES: 4

PREP TIME: 20 MINUTES

COOK TIME: 25 MINUTES

DUTCH BABY

6 tablespoons salted butter, divided

¾ cup buttermilk, room temperature

4 large eggs, room temperature

1½ teaspoons vanilla extract

3 tablespoons granulated sugar

¾ cup all-purpose flour

2 tablespoons powdered sugar for sprinkling

2 tablespoons butter for serving

LEMON-THYME BLUEBERRIES

¼ cup water

¼ cup maple syrup

Peel of one lemon

2 sprigs fresh thyme

1 cup blueberries

THE FIRST time I made a dutch baby, I was floored with how beautiful it was, all puffed and golden. That's not even the best part about this recipe. The *best part* is how simple it is. We all need more recipes like this in our lives. The ones that come together with a quick blitz of the blender and the magic of a piping-hot cast-iron skillet. These are the recipes that make us feel like superheroes in the kitchen. The whole family will be impressed, and no one ever needs to know how easy it was!

Preheat the oven to 450°F/230°C.

While the oven preheats, make the batter. Place 2 tablespoons of butter in a small bowl and microwave in 15-second intervals until melted. Add the buttermilk, eggs, vanilla extract, granulated sugar, and all-purpose flour to a blender. Blitz for 1 minute. With the blender running, slowly pour the melted butter into the batter. Let the batter stand for 10 minutes.

While the batter sets and once the oven is heated to temperature, place a large 12-inch cast-iron skillet in the oven for 10 minutes to get it screaming hot. At the 10-minute mark, add the remaining 3 tablespoons of butter to the hot skillet to melt, and leave it in the oven an additional 1–2 minutes.

Remove the heated skillet, pour the batter into the center, and quickly return to the oven. Bake for 20–25 minutes or until puffed and golden. Resist the urge to open the oven door, as it may deflate your dutch baby!

While the dutch baby bakes, make your Lemon-Thyme Blueberries. To a saucepan, add water, maple syrup, lemon peel, and thyme. Bring it to a simmer for 3 min-

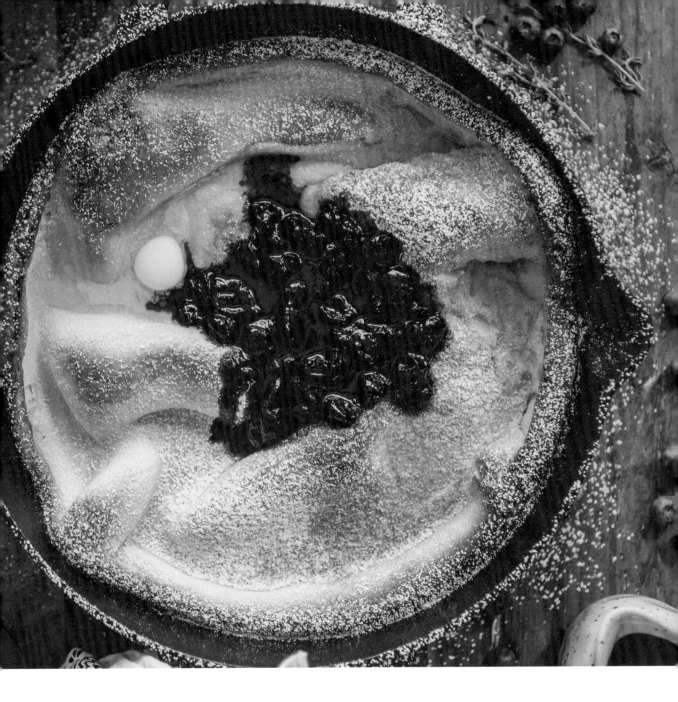

utes over medium-low heat. Remove the lemon peel and thyme sprigs. Add the blueberries and cook for 5–7 minutes until the berries are soft and bursting.

When the Dutch baby is complete, remove from the oven and sprinkle with powdered sugar. Top with the remaining butter and Lemon-Thyme Blueberries.

PECAN WAFFLES WITH MAPLE-BACON BUTTER

YIELDS: *6 WAFFLES*

PREP TIME: *20 MINUTES*

COOK TIME: *15–20 MINUTES*

1½ cups all-purpose flour

1 teaspoon salt

½ teaspoon baking soda

1 egg

½ cup plus 1 tablespoon granulated sugar

4 tablespoons butter, room temperature

¾ cup half-and-half

½ cup buttermilk

1 teaspoon vanilla

½ cup chopped pecans

Maple syrup for serving

ONE OF the Well-Fed Fraser's all-time favorite restaurants is a particular diner that specializes in waffles. The only reason to go to this special waffle diner is for their pecan waffles. We don't dine out often, but every now and then, after a big competition or during a long road trip, we stop for a stack covered in the "butter spread" and "pancake syrup." I was determined to bring that nostalgia home. No more butter spread on diner waffles!

In a medium bowl, whisk the flour, salt, and baking soda. Set aside.

In a large bowl, lightly beat the egg. Add the sugar and butter, mix well until smooth using a hand mixer. Add the half-and-half, buttermilk, and vanilla. Lastly, add the chopped pecans and mix with a silicone spatula.

Add the dry mix ingredients into the wet ingredients, mix with silicone spatula until just combined. Do not overmix. Place batter in the fridge to rest for 10 minutes while the waffle iron preheats.

Spray the waffle iron with cooking spray. Use a ¼ cup measuring cup to scoop batter into the center of the hot waffle iron.

Close the lid and cook for 3-4 minutes or until golden brown. Follow the cooking instructions for your particular waffle iron as cooking times may vary.

Remove the cooked waffle and place on a wire rack. Repeat the cooking steps; spray, scoop, and cook.

When ready to serve, spread with a generous serving of Maple-Bacon Butter and drizzle with maple syrup.

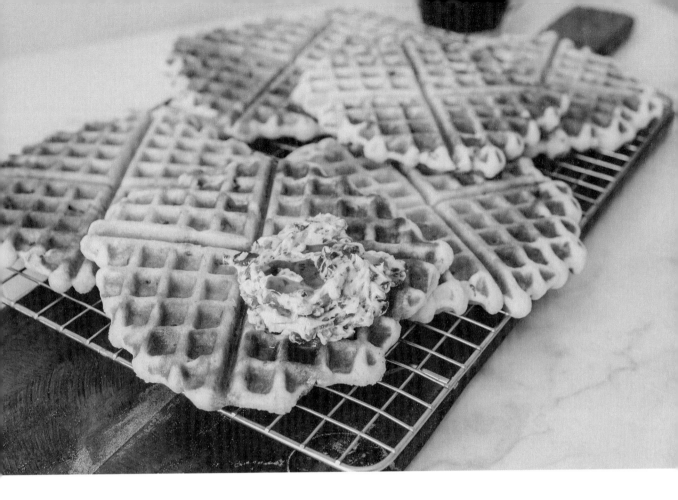

MAPLE-BACON BUTTER

YIELDS: 10-12 TABLESPOONS
PREP TIME: 10 MINUTES
COOK TIME: 0 MINUTES

½ cup (1 stick) salted butter, room temperature

3 slices bacon, cooked and diced

2 tablespoons maple syrup

NONE OF that "butter spread" around here. Serve with your waffles, pancakes, dutch babies, banana breads, and so on. The list goes on!

Place butter into the bowl of a stand mixer with the whisk attachment. Start the mixer on low, increase the speed to high, and whip butter until pale and fluffy, about 1–2 minutes.

With the mixer off, add the diced bacon and maple syrup. Whip until the ingredients are evenly combined. Use immediately or store in a mason jar in the fridge for future use.

BREAKFAST: SWEET

41

THE KING'S WAFFLE SAMMICH

SERVES: 4
PREP TIME: 10 MINUTES
COOK TIME: 20 MINUTES

8 slices thick-cut bacon

2 tablespoons maple syrup

4 leftover Pecan Waffles, cut in half

8 tablespoons almond butter

2 tablespoons honey

2 bananas, sliced

IF I'M going to turn on the waffle iron, I might as well double the batch and have a stock of waffles in the freezer for when the waffle craving hits. I also love to have a small stock of waffles around for when the bananas on the counter are perfectly ripe so I can whip up a sandwich made famous by the King, Elvis Presley. The combination of ingredients may seem a bit unlikely, but trust me on this one, it's a match made in heaven. Sweet and salty never disappoint, and this sandwich delivers not only on flavor but also on texture. While this varies just slightly from the King's original go-to recipe, the memory of it is kept alive.

Preheat the oven to 350°F/177°C. Drizzle the bacon with the maple syrup. Lay the strips of bacon on an aluminum foil-lined baking sheet. Bake for 15–20 minutes or until desired doneness. (We like it a little crispy!) Remove the bacon and place on a paper towel–lined plate. Once slightly cooled, tear each slice into 3–4 pieces and set aside.

Toast the waffle halves in the toaster. To each warmed waffle half, spread 1 tablespoon of almond butter. Drizzle a bit of honey over the almond butter and lay slices of banana on four waffle halves. Top the banana slices with bacon pieces, and top the sandwich with the remaining waffle halves. Serve immediately.

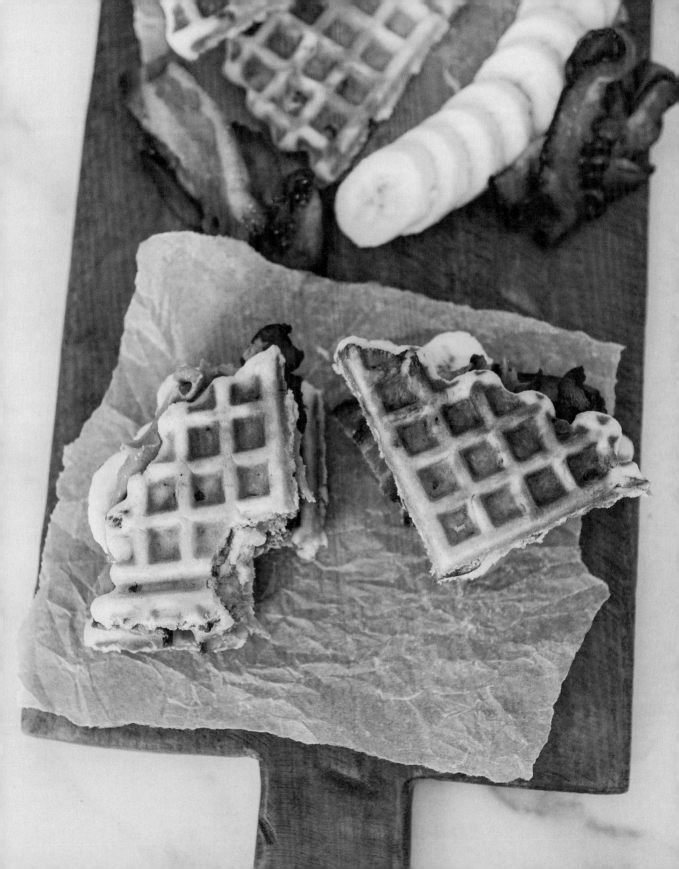

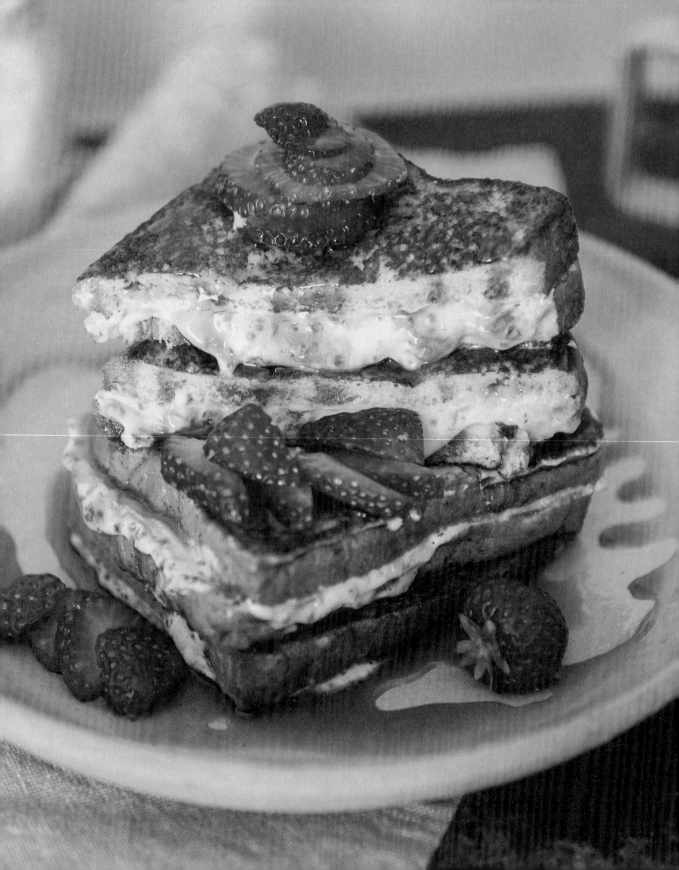

STRAWBERRIES & CREAM-STUFFED FRENCH TOAST

¼ cup water

¼ cup maple syrup

1 lemon peel

1 pint strawberries, sliced and divided

2 tablespoons chia seeds

8 ounces cream cheese, room temperature

4 eggs

½ cup whole milk (or heavy cream)

1 teaspoon cinnamon

1 teaspoon vanilla extract

8 slices brioche bread

4 teaspoons salted butter

Maple syrup for serving

I CANNOT take full credit for this recipe. The true creator of the cream cheese–stuffed french toast in our house is Mat. One morning, I had suggested peanut butter–stuffed french toast, and as he sat thinking about it, he wasn't immediately sold. He looked at me and asked, "Do we have any cream cheese?" The answer is always "YES" in this house, and the idea was born. I love topping pancakes and french toast with a combination of butter, syrup, and something fresh.

Combine the water, maple syrup, and lemon peel in a small saucepan over medium heat. Bring to low boil and reduce to simmer for 5 minutes. Remove the lemon peel. Add ¾ of the sliced strawberries and reserve the rest for serving. Cook on low heat for 5–7 minutes, stirring occasionally. Add the chia seeds, cook for an additional 5 minutes, then remove from the heat and place in a glass bowl to cool (yields about 1 cup).

Place the cream cheese in a small bowl and whip for 2 minutes using a hand mixer. Add 2 tablespoons of the cooled strawberry chia jam to the whipped cream cheese, swirl into the cream cheese with a spoon.

Whisk the eggs, milk, cinnamon, and vanilla in a shallow dish. To each slice of bread, evenly distribute the strawberry-swirled cream cheese. Pair two slices of bread together and dip the sandwich into the egg mixture, evenly coating both sides.

Add 1 teaspoon of butter to a nonstick skillet over medium heat. Cook each stuffed french toast for 2 minutes on each side. Cut in half, serve with reserved strawberry slices and maple syrup.

FRENCH TOAST BAGEL WITH HONEY-WALNUT WHIPPED CREAM CHEESE

1¾ cups warm water

4 tablespoons honey, divided

2 teaspoons dry active yeast

2 cups bread flour

2 cups whole-wheat flour

1½ teaspoons salt

1 tablespoon olive oil

3 eggs

1 teaspoon vanilla

1 tablespoon cinnamon, divided

2 tablespoons granulated sugar

Honey-Walnut Whipped Cream Cheese for serving (see recipe on page 48)

IF WE can dip plain bread into a cinnamon custard, then why not bagels? Warm cinnamon and sweet sugar all brought together with Honey-Walnut Whipped Cream Cheese. Bagels straight from the oven are a true treat, warm and steamy and no need to be toasted. These keep well stored in an airtight container for 3–4 days. Slice it in half, toast it up, and slather with sweet and nutty cream cheese to start your day off right.

Warm your water to 110°F/45°C. Pour ½ cup of the warm water into the bowl of a stand mixer. Add 2 tablespoons of honey and stir to help dissolve. Sprinkle the dry active yeast onto the top of the honey water and set aside for 5–10 minutes to bloom. The dry active yeast will bubble and foam.

In a large mixing bowl, measure flours and salt, stir to combine, and set aside.

Once the yeast has bloomed, add ½ of the flour mixture and with the dough hook attached begin to mix on low. Mix for 1 minute. Add the remaining flour and begin to pour the remaining water into the mixer as it works. Pour slowly and about a ¼ cup at a time. Allow the dry bits of flour to fully soak up the water before adding more. Knead the dough for 10 minutes until a smooth ball forms and pulls away from the sides of the bowl.

Remove the dough from the bowl. Pour olive oil into the bowl and use a paper towel to fully coat up the sides. Return the dough to the oiled bowl, cover with a damp kitchen towel, and place in a warm spot in the kitchen for at least an hour or until the dough has doubled in size.

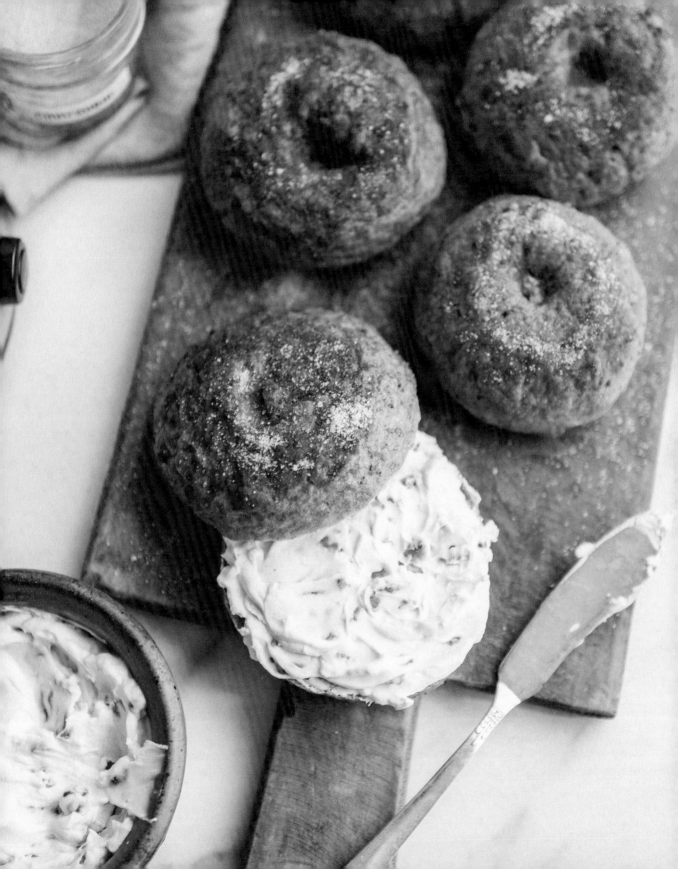

Punch the dough down to deflate it, cover it again, and let it rise another 30 minutes.

Turn the dough out onto a lightly floured surface. Knead for 2–3 minutes until smooth. Using a sharp knife, cut the dough into 8 sections. Smooth each section into a ball by pushing it into the counter with the palm of your hand while making a circular motion. Push your thumb through the center of the ball and work your hands around the dough to form your bagel shape. Place the dough onto a parchment-lined baking sheet. Allow to rise for 20 minutes.

When ready to bake, preheat the oven to 425°F/220°C. Bring a large pot of water to a rolling boil and add the remaining 2 tablespoons of honey to the water bath. In a shallow dish, whisk the eggs, vanilla, and 2 teaspoons of cinnamon, set aside. In a separate small dish, combine remaining 1 teaspoon of cinnamon and 2 tablespoons of granulated sugar, and set aside.

Boil each bagel for 1 minute on each side, and place boiled bagels on a sheet of parchment paper. Dip each bagel into the egg wash mixture and cover all sides. Place the dipped bagels on a dry parchment-lined baking sheet. Sprinkle the bagels with the cinnamon-sugar mixture. Bake at 425°F/220°C for 18–20 minutes until golden.

Remove the bagels from the oven, let cool on the baking sheet for 2 minutes, and then move to a wire rack. Either let the bagels completely cool and store in an airtight container, or consume immediately while warm with Honey-Walnut Whipped Cream Cheese.

HONEY-WALNUT WHIPPED CREAM CHEESE

YIELDS: 1¼ CUP
PREP TIME: 3-5 MINUTES
COOK TIME: 0 MINUTES

8 oz. cream cheese, room temperature

2 tablespoons plus 1 teaspoon honey

¼ cup raw walnuts, finely chopped

In a medium bowl, whip the room-temperature cream cheese using a hand mixer (or stand mixer) until fluffy, about 2 minutes. Add the honey and whip for an additional minute. Gently fold in the walnuts using a silicone spatula and serve with French Toast Bagel (or use in Mini Stone Fruit Tarts on page 194).

CORN, CREAM CHEESE & BLACKBERRY SWIRL MUFFINS

YIELDS: 12 MUFFINS
PREP TIME: 15 MINUTES
COOK TIME: 18 MINUTES

1 cup all-purpose flour

1 cup cornmeal

½ teaspoon salt

¼ teaspoon baking soda

1½ teaspoons baking powder

½ cup salted butter, melted

½ cup granulated sugar

¾ cup buttermilk

1 large egg

4 ounces cream cheese, room temperature

1 tablespoon honey

¼ cup Blackberry-Chia Jam (see page 54 for recipe)

FOOD EXPERIENCES bring in all the senses, not just taste. I think we love these muffins so much for the textures as much as the taste. Slightly sweet cornmeal that crunches with each bite pairs with soft and tangy cream cheese and fresh pops of blackberries. When it is morning and time to wake up, these muffins will do the trick!

Preheat the oven to 400°F/200°C. Prepare a muffin tin with muffin paper liners and set aside.

Whisk the flour, cornmeal, salt, baking soda, and baking powder in a medium mixing bowl.

In a separate large mixing bowl, whisk the melted butter, granulated sugar, buttermilk, and egg until fully combined. In two batches, mix the dry ingredients into the large mixing bowl of wet ingredients.

In a small bowl, whisk the room temperature cream cheese and honey until smooth.

Scoop the batter into a prepared muffin tin until the muffin cups are ⅔ of the way full. Add 1–2 teaspoons of the cream cheese mixture and 1–2 teaspoons of Blackberry-Chia Jam to each muffin. Use a toothpick or skewer to swirl each muffin slightly.

Bake for 15–18 minutes or until the muffins are golden brown. Transfer muffin tin to a cooling rack for 5 minutes.

Remove the muffins from the tin and cool an additional 5 minutes before serving.

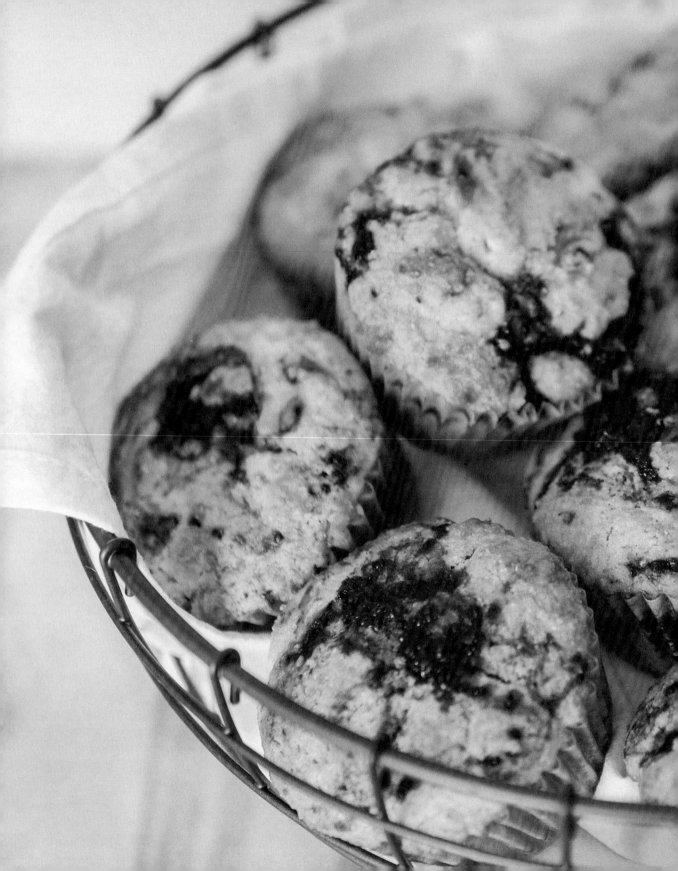

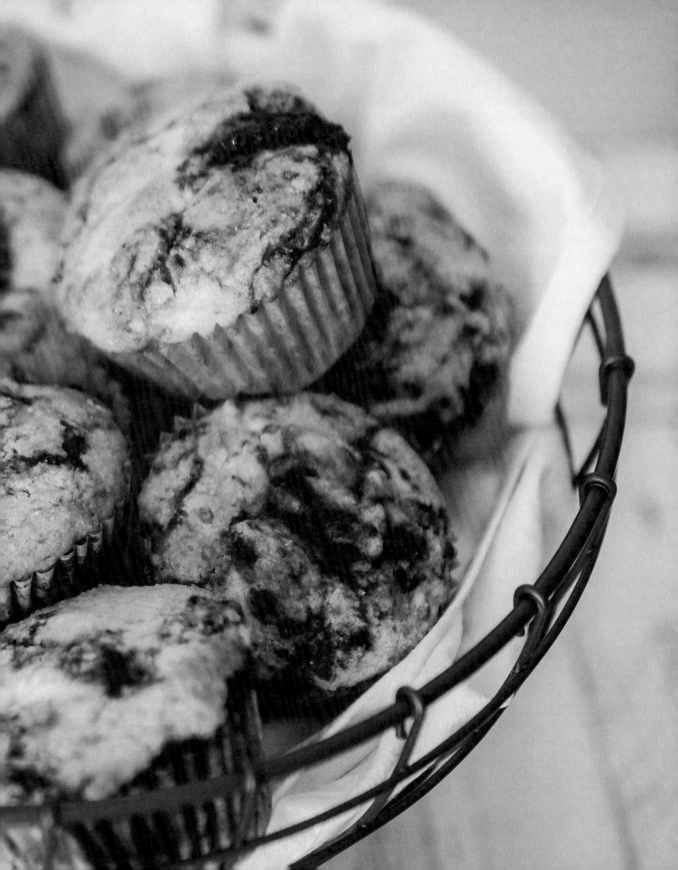

HICKORY-SMOKED PECAN GRANOLA

SERVES: *12*

PREP TIME: *35 MINUTES*

COOK TIME: *35 MINUTES*

2 cups old-fashioned oats

1 cup steel-cut oats

¼ cup pumpkin seeds

¼ cup hazelnuts, chopped

¾ cup pecans, chopped

1 teaspoon cinnamon

½ teaspoon cardamom

¼ cup maple syrup

½ cup olive oil

½ cup light brown sugar

1½ teaspoons pure vanilla extract

1 egg white

1–2 pinches flaky salt

I KNOW not everyone has a smoker at home, and it would be silly of me to put it on your list of kitchen essentials. That's just not realistic! Fear not! These recipes have been tested on the smoker as well as in the oven, and the temperature and times are the same. Will you be missing that hint of smoke? Yes. Will it ruin the food experience of this recipe? No. Don't sweat it! The sweet smell of toasted pecans and maple syrup will fill your home, and you'll be so consumed with eagerness to taste test these yummy clusters of granola you won't even notice the difference. For those of you who have a smoker, get your hands on some hickory pellets or chips and bask in that wood-fired flavor.

Preheat the Traeger Grill (or oven) to 200°F/93°C.

In a large bowl, mix the old-fashioned oats, steel-cut oats, pumpkin seeds, hazelnuts, pecans, cinnamon, and cardamom.

In a separate small bowl, whisk maple syrup, olive oil, light brown sugar, vanilla extract, and egg white. Pour the wet ingredients into the bowl of dry ingredients and mix well to fully coat the oats.

Lay the oat mixture onto a parchment-lined baking sheet. Pat down to compact. Sprinkle with flaky salt. Place the baking sheet directly on the preheated grill, close the lid, and bake for 15 minutes. Remove from the grill, toss, and pat down again.

Increase the grill temperature to 300°F/150°C. Return the granola to the grill for an additional 20 minutes.

Allow the granola to cool for 30 minutes before touching; this will help form clusters. Store in an airtight container. Serve with yogurt and fresh berries or eat like a bowl of cereal with cold milk of choice!

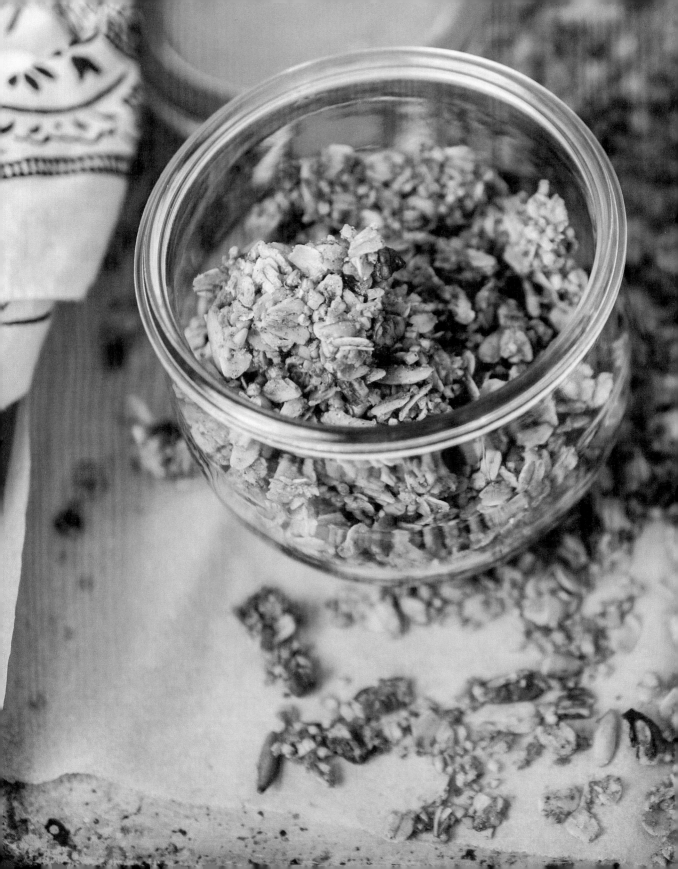

BLACKBERRY & PEAR OVERNIGHT OATS

SERVES: 4
*PREP TIME: 5 MINUTES (PLUS
4–24 HOURS)*
COOK TIME: 0 MINUTES

OATS

2 cups full-fat coconut milk

1 cup greek yogurt

3 tablespoons maple syrup

1 tablespoon chia seeds

1 teaspoon vanilla extract

½ teaspoon cardamom

¼ teaspoon cinnamon

¼ teaspoon salt

2 cups old-fashioned rolled oats

2 pears, sliced for serving

BLACKBERRY-CHIA JAM

¼ cup water

¼ cup maple syrup

1 lemon peel

2 cups blackberries (fresh or frozen)

2 tablespoons chia seeds

SOMETIMES YOU just need a quick bite in the morning or something to curb a midnight sweet tooth. This is a great go-to recipe for any time of the day. Easy to prep *and* easy to make substitutions with what you have on hand. If you prefer to use regular milk instead of coconut milk, swap it out! If you want to make it dairy-free, exchange the greek yogurt with your choice of dairy-free yogurt. You've got frozen blueberries instead of blackberries? Easy swap! The only ingredient that must stay is the rolled oats; they are the best option for soaking. Save the steel-cut and quick-cook oats for your warm bowls of porridge.

In a large bowl, whisk the coconut milk, greek yogurt, maple syrup, chia seeds, vanilla, cardamom, cinnamon, and salt until smooth. Add the rolled oats and stir to combine. Cover and refrigerate for at least 2 hours, but ideally overnight. To make the Blackberry-Chia Jam, add the water, maple syrup, and lemon peel to a small saucepan over medium heat. Bring to low boil and reduce to simmer for 5 minutes. Remove the lemon peel and add the blackberries. Cook on low heat for 5–7 minutes, stirring occasionally, until the berries are bursting (you will need to cook longer if using frozen). Add the chia seeds, cook for an additional 5 minutes, then remove from the heat and place in a glass bowl to cool (yields about 1 cup).

When ready to serve, top the chilled overnight oats with a dollop or two of Blackberry-Chia Jam and sliced pears.

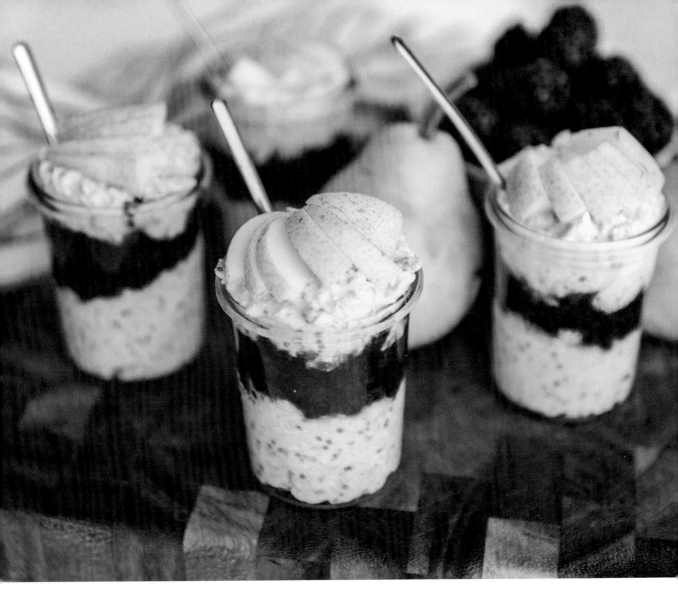

PRO TIP

Portion out into 4 individual servings using mason jars before chilling in the refrigerator; it makes for easy grab-and-go mornings.

CARROT CAKE STEEL-CUT OATS WITH CREAM CHEESE YOGURT & HONEY GLAZED PECANS

SERVES: 10–12
PREP TIME: 15 MINUTES
COOK TIME: 6–8 HOURS

OATS

2½ cups steel-cut oats

¼ cup shredded coconut

1 cup shredded carrots

5 cups water

2½ cups canned full-fat coconut milk

1 cup pineapple juice

½ cup maple syrup

1½ teaspoons cinnamon

1 teaspoon ginger

¼ teaspoon ground nutmeg

¼ teaspoon ground cloves

1 teaspoon vanilla extract

HONEY GLAZED PECANS

1 cup raw pecans, chopped

¼ cup honey

2 tablespoons canned full-fat coconut milk

1 tablespoon flaky salt

CREAM CHEESE YOGURT TOPPING

4 ounces cream cheese, room temperature

1 cup vanilla greek yogurt

2 tablespoons maple syrup

THIS IS my go-to for when we have houseguests. It packs a ton of flavor and feeds a crowd. I have made this in both the pressure cooker and the slow cooker. If you're using a slow cooker, the ideal size for overnight 6–8 hours of cooking is a 3-quart pot. If you're using a 6-plus quart pot, the cook time will be 2–3 hours. When using a pressure cooker, you must allow the cooker to naturally release for at least 20 minutes. There is foam generated when cooking oats that could potentially clog the pressure-release vent.

Generously spray the bottom and sides of the pressure cooker with cooking spray. Mix all the ingredients for the oatmeal into the bowl of the pressure cooker. Cover and cook on high for 10 minutes. When the pressure cook has completed, allow the pressure cooker to naturally release for 20 minutes. At the 20-minute mark, move the pressure knob to *vent* to release any remaining pressure. Remove the lid and stir the oats.

To make the Honey Glazed Pecans, heat a skillet over medium-low heat, add the pecans, and toast 3–4 minutes. Add the honey and stir. Add the coconut milk and cook until it resembles a caramel, about 3 minutes. Remove the pan from the heat, lay the pecans on a parchment-lined baking sheet, sprinkle with flaky sea salt, and cool.

Before serving, mix the softened cream cheese, yogurt, and maple syrup.

To serve, scoop the oats into a bowl and top with a dollop or two of the yogurt and a handful of the honey and sea salt pecans.

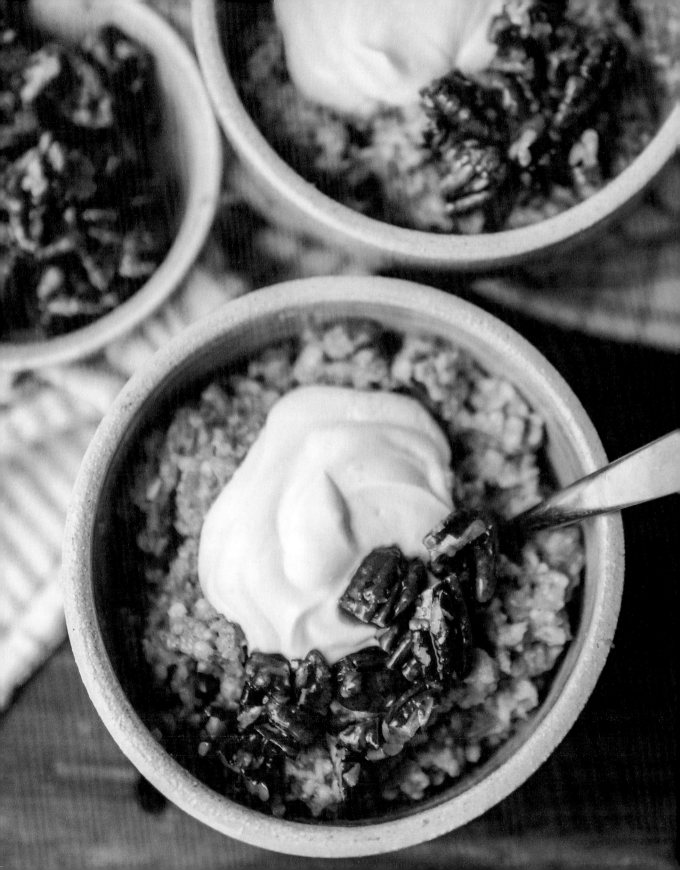

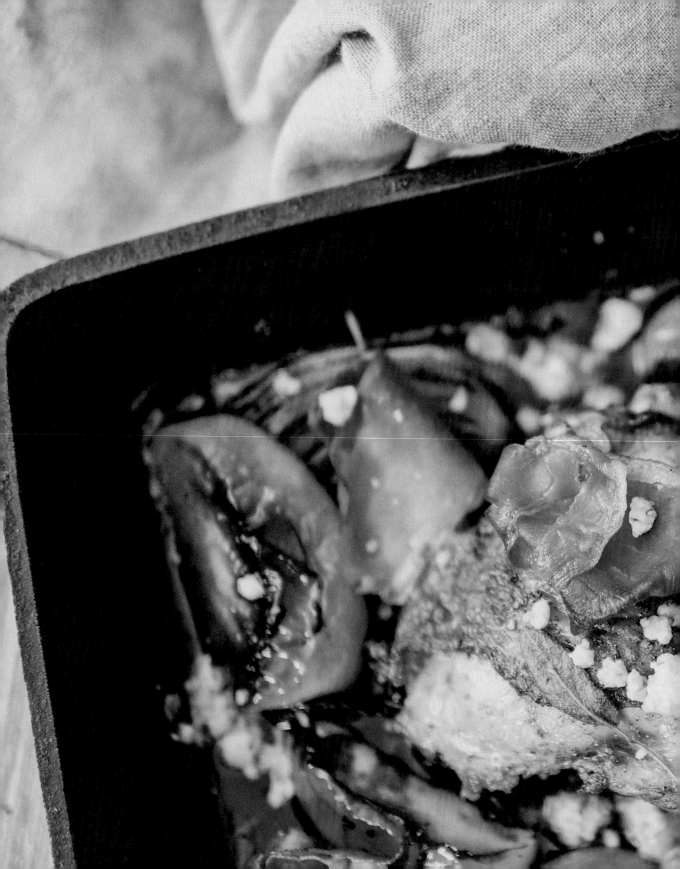

POULTRY
& PORK

PIRI PIRI CHICKEN WINGS & YOGURT DIPPING SAUCE

SERVES: *4*
PREP TIME: *10 MINUTES*
COOK TIME: *25 MINUTES*

PIRI PIRI SAUCE

4 cloves garlic

¼ cup dried Thai chilies, rehydrated

½ cup jarred roasted red peppers, drained

1 teaspoon smoked paprika

½ cup fresh cilantro leaves

¼ cup fresh basil leaves

¼ cup olive oil

1 lemon, juiced

Salt to taste

CHICKEN WINGS

3 pounds party wings

1 teaspoon salt

1 teaspoon pepper

1 teaspoon garlic powder

YOGURT DIPPING SAUCE

½ cup plain greek yogurt

1 teaspoon cumin

1 teaspoon lemon juice

2 tablespoons cilantro leaves, chopped

IF YOU do not have an air fryer of any kind, you can absolutely make these in the oven. Pat the wings dry with a paper towel; do not skip this step if you want crispy skins. When you season the wings with salt, pepper, and garlic powder, also add 2 teaspoons of baking powder. Place the wings on a baking rack over a baking sheet to make sure the hot air is circulating around the wings for an even cook and crisp. Bake at 425°F/220°C for 40–50 minutes or until internal temperature reaches 165°F, and always sauce after you bake for the best crisp.

With the food processor running, toss the cloves of garlic into the chute; this will help break them down into small bits. Turn the food processor off, add the remaining Piri Piri Sauce ingredients. Blitz until smooth. Taste and add salt as needed. This sauce yields 12 ounces. Store it in an airtight jar in the refrigerator (use leftover sauce to make Roasted Cod, Bursting Summer Tomatoes, Sweet Corn & Crispy Prosciutto on page 119).

Place the wings in a large bowl, sprinkle with salt, pepper, and garlic powder. Toss until evenly coated. Place wings in the basket of the air fryer, working in batches depending on the size of the basket. Set the temperature to 400°F/200°C and crisp the wings for 20 minutes, checking halfway to toss and rearrange the wings. Once the wings have reached an internal temperature of 165°F/73°C, remove them from the air fryer.

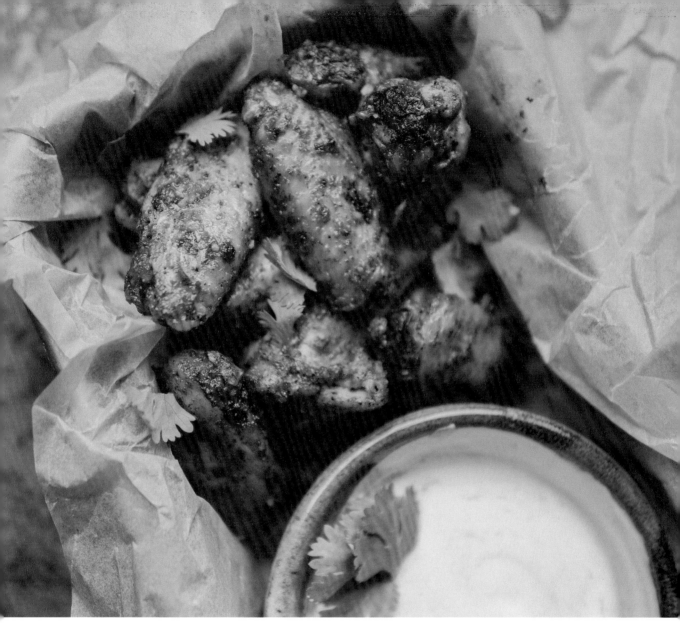

Toss the wings in 2–4 tablespoons of the Piri Piri (more if you like saucy and spicy wings!), return the wings to the basket, and crisp an additional 2–4 minutes to allow the sauce to caramelize.

Just before serving, mix the greek yogurt, cumin, lemon juice, and cilantro leaves. Serve the wings with the yogurt dipping sauce.

MAPLE MUSTARD SPATCHCOCK CHICKEN

SERVES: 4–6
PREP TIME: 24 HOURS
COOK TIME: 60 MINUTES

BRINE

2 quarts water

⅓ cup kosher salt

1 lemon, quartered

10 sprigs fresh parsley

3 dried bay leaves

¼ cup maple syrup

6 garlic cloves, smashed

1 tablespoon black peppercorns

SPATCHCOCK CHICKEN

1 (4–6 pound) whole chicken

2 teaspoons kosher salt

2 teaspoons ground black pepper

2 teaspoons garlic powder

¼ cup maple syrup

¼ cup salted butter, melted

2 tablespoons dijon mustard

2 teaspoons apple cider vinegar

1 teaspoon worcestershire sauce

SPATCHCOCK CHICKEN must have been the first "chefy" thing I learned how to do, and you can bet if we have a whole bird in the house, I'm going to spatchcock it. To spatchcock means to cut the backbone out and lay the bird flat, cut-side down. This ensures a more even cook. Less worry about the chicken thighs being overdone while the chicken breast is still pink. Grab your kitchen shears and let's get cooking!

Add 2 cups of water, kosher salt, quartered lemon, parsley, bay leaves, maple syrup, smashed garlic cloves, and peppercorns to a large pot. Bring to a boil to dissolve the salt, and then remove from the heat. Add the remaining water to cool the pot. Cool completely before using (about 1 hour).

Fully submerge the chicken in the brine and refrigerate for 12–24 hours. Remove from the brine, pat dry, and prep the chicken for cooking. Spatchcock the bird by cutting out the spine with a pair of kitchen scissors.

Preheat the Traeger Grill to 450°F/230°C. Place the chicken cut-side down on a baking sheet. Season with salt, pepper, and garlic powder. When the grill reaches temperature, place the chicken cut-side down directly on the grill grates. Cook for 45 minutes.

In a small bowl, whisk the maple syrup, melted butter, dijon mustard, apple cider vinegar, and worcestershire sauce. Brush the chicken 2–3 times within the remaining cook time (about 15–25 minutes depending on size) until the internal temperature reaches 165°F/73°C. Remove the chicken from the grill, brush with any remaining glaze, and rest for 10–15 minutes before cutting into the chicken.

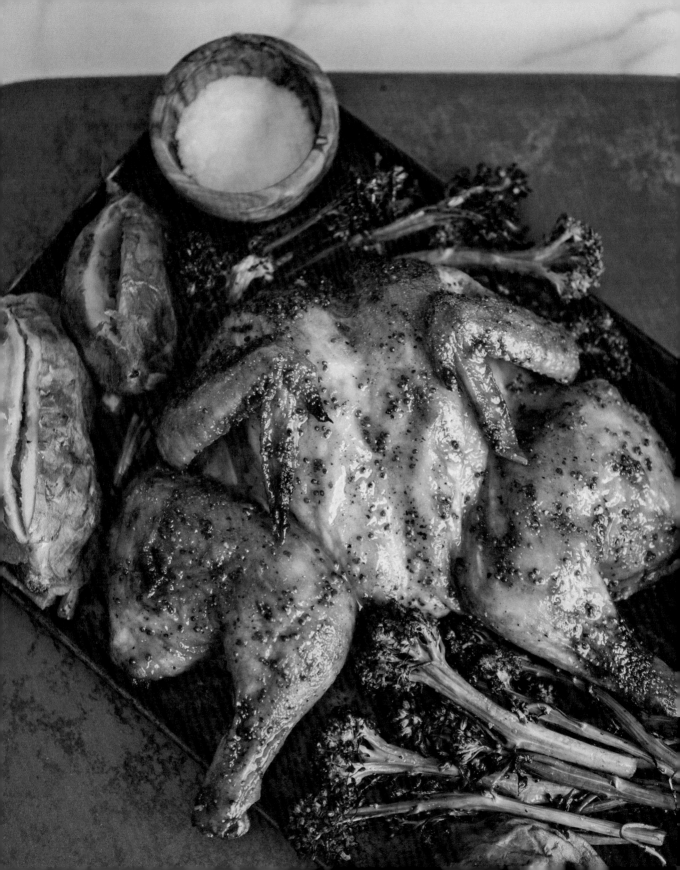

SPICED CHICKEN WITH GREEN SAUCE

SERVES: 4

PREP TIME: 30 MINUTES (PLUS 4–24 HOURS MARINATING)

COOK TIME: 40 MINUTES

4 garlic cloves, minced

2 tablespoons olive oil

2 tablespoons lime juice

2 teaspoons honey

1 tablespoon cumin

2 teaspoons smoked paprika

1 teaspoon coriander

1 teaspoon oregano

1½ teaspoons kosher salt

1 teaspoon soy sauce (tamari or liquid aminos)

8 boneless, skin-on chicken thighs

1 tablespoon olive oil

WE ALL want simple dinners, amiright? Marinate your chicken overnight or whip it together in the morning before work, and thank your prepared self later. The greatest part about this meal is that it can all be prepped the day before and stored in the fridge until you're ready to cook the chicken. It comes together quickly and packs a ton of flavor. No need for boring meals! Great served with Grilled Corn & Cucumber Salad.

In a large bowl, whisk the first ten ingredients to make the marinade. Add the chicken thighs to the bowl, turning over in the marinade to cover all sides. Cover with plastic wrap and place in the fridge for a minimum of 4 hours up to overnight.

Preheat the oven to 350°F/177°C. While the oven comes up to temperature, remove the chicken from the fridge and sit it on the counter for 30 minutes to remove the chill.

Heat a cast-iron skillet over medium-high heat with olive oil. When the oil shimmers, add the chicken skin-side down. Brown chicken on each side 3–4 minutes.

Place the skillet in the oven to finish cooking the chicken until the internal temperature reaches 165°F/73°C, about 10–15 minutes. Remove the skillet from the oven. Rest the chicken 5 minutes before plating. Serve the chicken with steamed white rice drizzled with Green Sauce and Grilled Corn & Cucumber Salad (see page 158 for recipe).

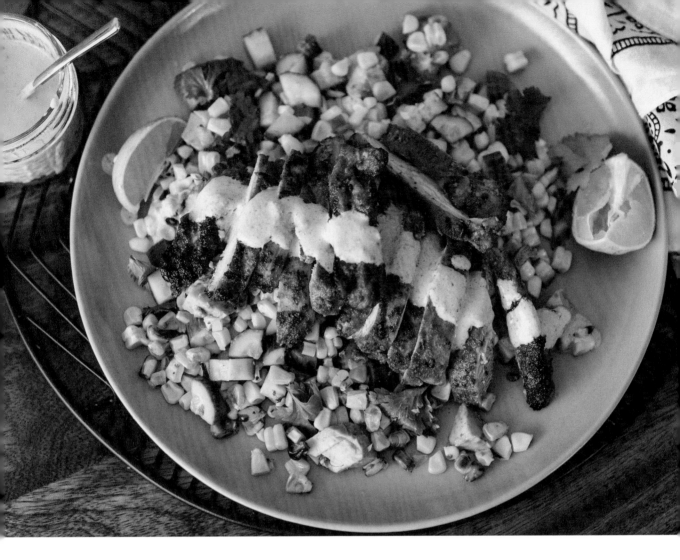

GREEN SAUCE

SERVES: 4
PREP TIME: 5 MINUTES
COOK TIME: 0 MINUTES

½ cup plain Skyr
½ jalapeño, seeded
1 garlic clove
1 cup cilantro
2 tablespoons lime juice
Salt to taste

I LIKE using Skyr or greek yogurt for this sauce because it's very thick and gives a great consistency to the sauce.

Place all ingredients in a blender. Pulse 3–5 times, then set the blender to high. Blend until smooth, about 1 minute. Pour green sauce into a mason jar, cover, and chill until ready to serve.

SPINACH-ARTICHOKE CHICKEN PICCATA

SERVES: 4
PREP TIME: 10 MINUTES
COOK TIME: 30 MINUTES

4–6 chicken breasts, butterflied

Salt and pepper to taste

1 cup white cornmeal

8 tablespoons salted butter, divided

1 pound angel hair pasta

⅓ cup lemon juice

3–4 thin lemon slices

⅓ cup white wine (or chicken stock)

⅓ cup heavy cream

¼ cup capers, drained and rinsed

1 (15-ounce) jar marinated artichoke heart halves, drained and roughly chopped

1 cup fresh baby spinach

Fresh chopped parsley for serving

LEMONY, TANGY, and creamy pasta. Perfectly browned chicken cutlets with a slight crunch to the breading. Fresh spinach and lightly marinated artichokes. My mouth is watering just listing the ingredients! It's not often you'll find pasta on the dinner table in our house, but when we do, it's something complex in flavor yet simple to make.

Pat the chicken dry with a paper towel. Season to taste with salt and pepper.

Place the white cornmeal in a shallow bowl. Dredge each piece of chicken in the cornmeal, shake off excess, and move to a separate clean plate.

Heat a large skillet over medium heat. Add 2 tablespoons of butter to the skillet and cook until foamy and fragrant. Working in two batches, lay the first batch of chicken in a single layer in the pan, leaving a little room between each to allow for crisping. Cook for 5–7 minutes on each side, depending on the thickness of each cutlet. Remove the chicken from the pan and set aside on a clean plate. Repeat this process with the remaining chicken.

While the second batch of chicken is cooking, bring a large pot of salted water to a boil. Place the pasta in the pot and cook to package instructions or to desired doneness (we like al dente!). Before straining the pasta, reserve 1 cup of pasta water. Do not rinse the pasta. Set aside.

To the hot chicken skillet, add the remaining 4 tablespoons of butter, use a wooden spoon to swirl the butter and pick up the brown bits on the bottom of the pan. Cook the butter until frothy and browned. To the butter, add lemon juice, lemon slices, white wine, heavy cream,

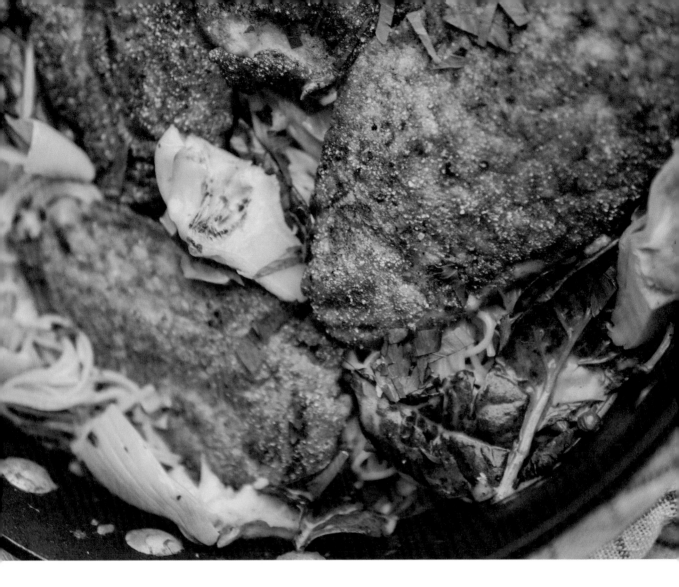

and capers. Stirring quickly to incorporate, reduce the heat to low and simmer for 2–3 minutes. Turn the heat off.

Add the cooked pasta directly to the sauce, twirling the pasta using tongs to fully coat. Add the artichokes and spinach; the residual heat from the sauce and pasta will lightly wilt the spinach. Use the reserved pasta water, 1–2 tablespoons, at this time to thin the sauce if needed.

Return the cooked chicken to the pan. Serve whole or slice the chicken before adding to the pan. Top with freshly chopped parsley and enjoy!

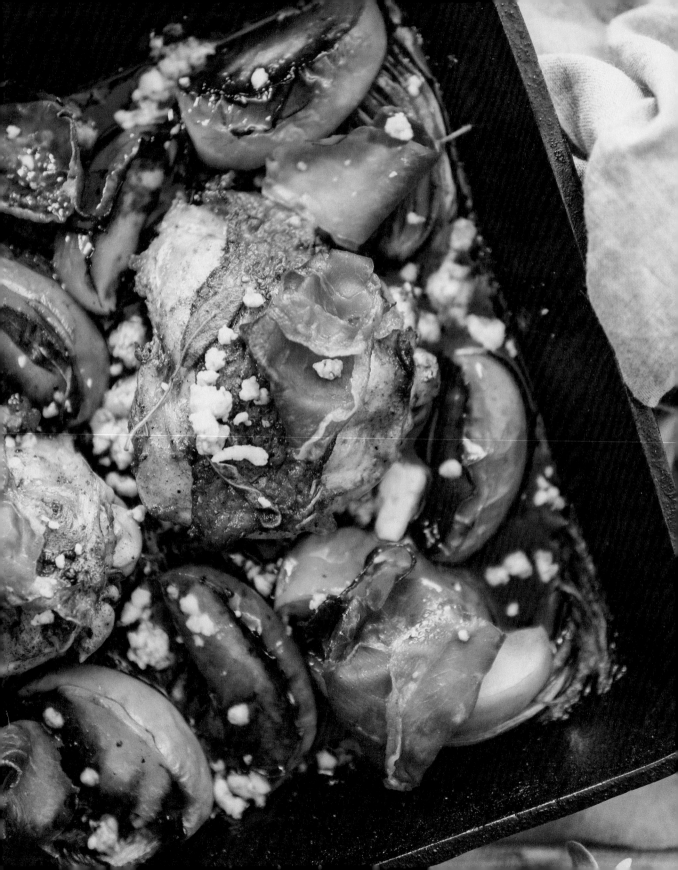

HONEYCRISP & BLUE CHEESE CHICKEN SKILLET

SERVES: 4

PREP TIME: 5 MINUTES

COOK TIME: 40 MINUTES

4 tablespoons salted butter

6 bone-in, skin-on chicken thighs

1 teaspoon ground sage

1 teaspoon kosher salt

½ teaspoon freshly ground pepper

2 tablespoons sherry vinegar

1 tablespoon honey

1 large sweet onion, thickly sliced

2 honeycrisp apples, thickly sliced

4–6 fresh sage leaves

8 ounces prosciutto

4 ounces blue cheese crumbles for serving

YOU MIGHT be thinking, *Sammy—apples, blue cheese, and chicken? I don't think that's going to work.* You're not alone! Mat said those exact words to me. I asked him to try it. To trust me. He did, and here it is in this book. It may sound like an odd combination, but oddly enough, it works and it's delicious! Sweet apples, salty bold cheese, and crisp lightly herbed chicken skins. Bold flavors and ready in 40 minutes, this is a new weeknight go-to!

Preheat the oven to high broil.

Heat a large cast-iron skillet over medium heat. Add the salted butter and cook until frothy and fragrant, about 2 minutes.

Pat the chicken dry with paper towels and season with the ground sage, salt, and pepper. Place the chicken, skin-side down, into the hot butter. Cook for 3–5 minutes on each side until deep golden brown. Move the chicken from the skillet to rest on a plate.

Return the skillet to the stove over medium heat. To the pan drippings, add the sherry vinegar and honey. Stir to combine using a wooden spoon to pick up any browned bits on the bottom of the skillet. Add the thickly sliced onion to the skillet. Reduce the heat to low and cook for 7–10 minutes until lightly caramelized. Add the apples and fresh sage to the skillet and toss to coat.

Return the chicken to the skillet and place in the preheated oven. Cook for an additional 7–10 minutes or until the internal temperature of the chicken reaches 165°F/73°C. In the last two minutes of cooking, top the skillet with curls of prosciutto. Remove the skillet from the oven, sprinkle with blue cheese, and serve.

POULTRY & PORK

ROASTED GARLIC-PARMESAN DRUMSTICKS

SERVES: 4
PREP TIME: 10 MINUTES
COOK TIME: 75 MINUTES

2 garlic bulbs

3 tablespoons olive oil, divided

3 pounds chicken drumsticks

1 tablespoon garlic powder

2 teaspoons salt

2 teaspoons black pepper

½ cup mayo

1 tablespoon dijon mustard

⅓ cup Parmesan cheese, grated, plus more for serving

1 teaspoon lemon juice

1 tablespoon apple cider vinegar

¼ teaspoon thyme

¼ teaspoon oregano

½ teaspoon red pepper flakes

Salt and pepper to taste

Fresh parsley, roughly chopped for garnish

GARLIC PARMESAN, a classic flavor combination and a household favorite. Saucy, cheesy, and popping with fresh herbs, it keeps you coming back for more. Serve alongside a light salad, simple steamed vegetables, and rice for a complete meal—or stack your plate high and snack on these while watching your favorite sports team hit the field. Your house, your rules!

Preheat the oven to 400°F/200°C.

Cut the tops off the garlic bulbs to expose the cloves. Place the bulbs on a square of aluminum foil, pour a tablespoon of olive oil on each, and wrap tightly. Roast in the oven for 40–45 minutes or until the cloves are soft and caramelized.

While the garlic roasts, heat a cast-iron skillet with a tablespoon of olive oil over medium-high heat. Season the drumsticks with garlic powder, salt, and pepper. Sear the chicken 2-3 minutes on all sides.

When the garlic is done roasting, remove the garlic skin and place the cloves in the bowl of a food processor with the remaining ingredients. Blitz on high for 1 minute or until smooth.

Remove the cast-iron skillet from the heat, pour half of the garlic-Parmesan mixture into the skillet, toss well. Place the skillet in the oven for 15–20 minutes or until the internal temperature of the chicken reaches 165°F/73°C. Pour the remaining garlic-Parmesan mixture into the cast-iron skillet and toss to combine. Sprinkle the drumsticks with fresh parsley and Parmesan before serving.

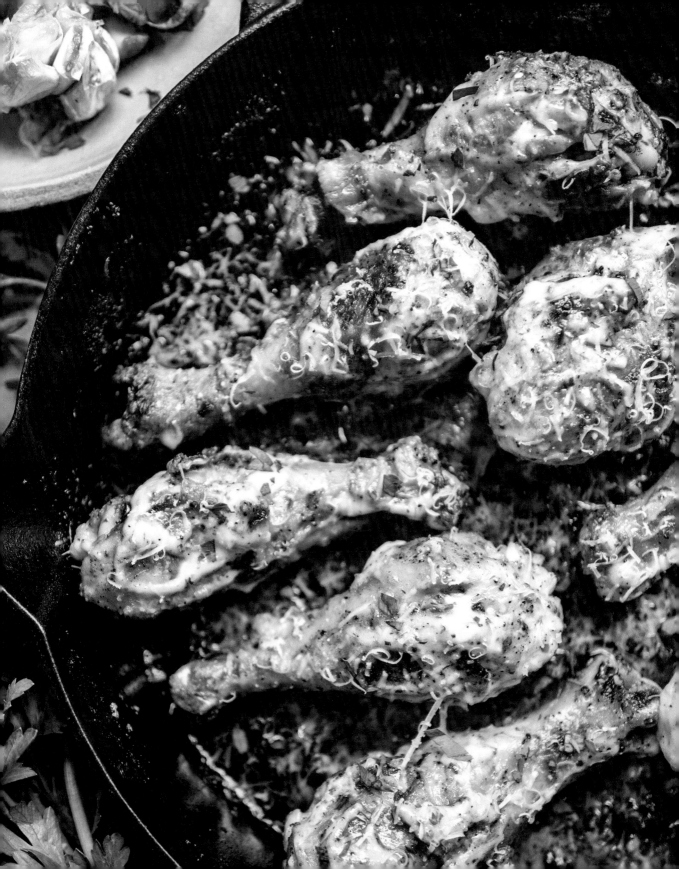

COCONUT-CURRY CHICKEN-STUFFED SWEET POTATOES

SERVES: 4–6

PREP TIME: 10 MINUTES

COOK TIME: 40 MINUTES

4–6 medium sweet potatoes

4 boneless, skinless chicken breasts

4 ounces shiitake mushrooms, sliced

4 ounces cremini mushrooms, sliced

1 cup low-sodium chicken broth

1 (14-ounce) can coconut milk

2 tablespoons low-sodium soy sauce

1 tablespoon fish sauce

1 tablespoon honey

⅓ cup creamy peanut butter

¼ cup Thai red curry paste

1-inch piece fresh ginger, grated

2 cloves garlic, minced or grated

¼ cup lime juice

2 teaspoons toasted sesame oil for serving

¼ cup cilantro, roughly chopped, for serving

1 red chili, sliced, for serving

2 green onions, sliced, for serving

Lime wedges for serving

LOADED BAKED potatoes just got outdone with these Coconut-Curry Chicken–Stuffed Sweet Potatoes. Not sure I could ever go back to the old-school plain baked potato with traditional fixings. I've lived life on the flavor edge, and now any less just isn't worth the space in my stomach. These stuffed sweet potatoes are great for meal prep and will keep you and your family well-fed.

Preheat the oven to 425°F/220°C.

Poke a handful of holes into the skin of each sweet potato and wrap with aluminum foil. Place the wrapped potatoes on a baking sheet and bake in the preheated oven for 30–40 minutes until tender. Remove from the oven and set aside until ready to serve.

While the sweet potatoes bake, prepare the chicken. To the bowl of the pressure cooker, add the chicken, shiitake mushrooms, and cremini mushrooms. In a large bowl, whisk the chicken broth, coconut milk, soy sauce, fish sauce, honey, peanut butter, curry paste, ginger, and garlic. Pour the liquid over the chicken and mushrooms. Mix to fully coat.

Place the pressure cook lid on and be sure to check the vent is closed. Set the pressure cooker to high for 10 minutes. When the cook is complete, allow the pressure to release naturally for 5 minutes and then do a quick release.

Remove the lid, take the chicken out, and place on a cutting board or baking sheet. Shred the chicken with two forks and return the shredded chicken to the pot. Add the lime juice and stir.

Cut a slice down the center of the sweet potato about halfway through the potato. Use a fork to open the cut and lightly mash the potato in its skin to make room for the shredded chicken filling.

Fill each potato with a heaping scoop of chicken and mushrooms. Drizzle each potato with a little toasted sesame oil and top with cilantro, red chili, green onions, and an extra squeeze of lime juice.

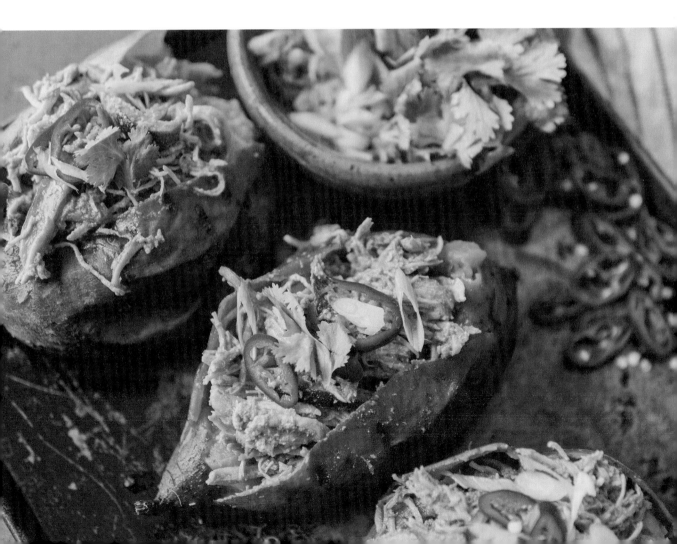

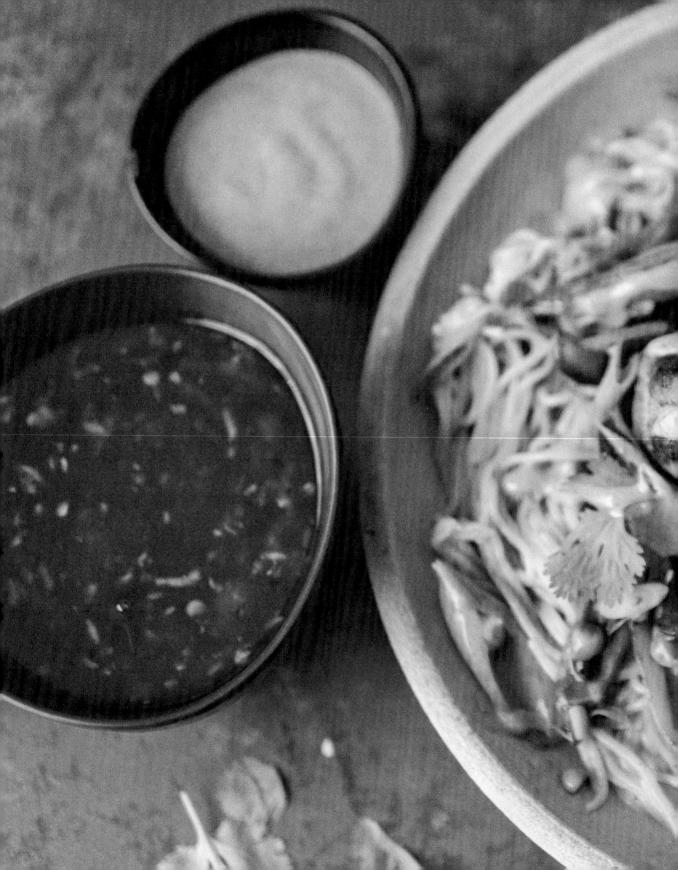

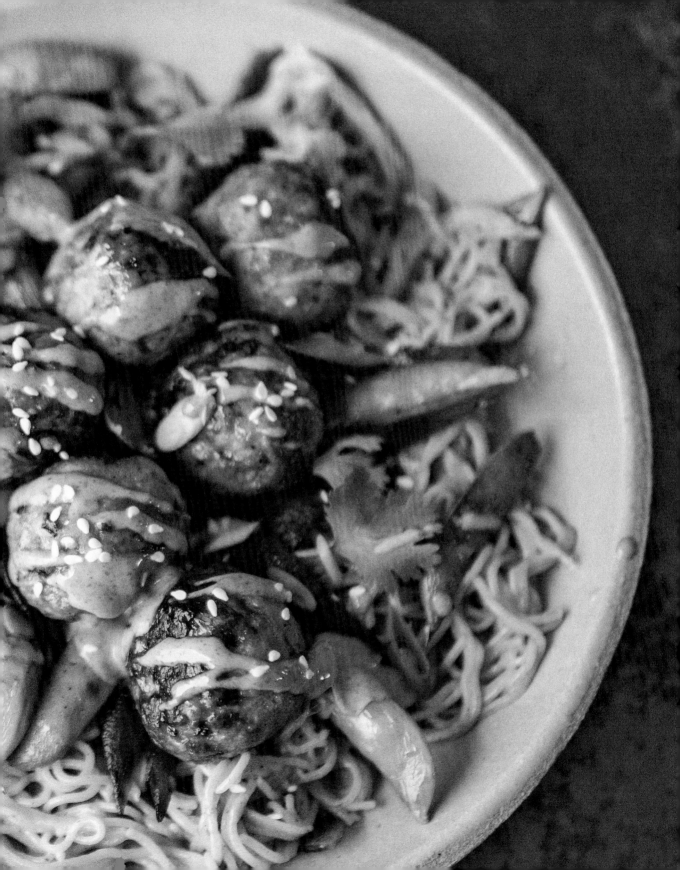

SWEET CHILI MEATBALL STIR-FRY

SERVES: 4
PREP TIME: 35 MINUTES
COOK TIME: 25 MINUTES

1 pound ground turkey (or chicken!)

½ pound ground pork

⅓ cup scallions, minced, plus more for garnish

2 tablespoons cilantro leaves, chopped, plus more for garnish

1 tablespoon fresh ginger, grated

2 garlic cloves, grated

2 teaspoons toasted sesame oil

2 teaspoons tamari

1 teaspoon fish sauce

1½ cups panko

¼ cup Sweet Chili Sauce (recipe on the following page)

1 tablespoon olive oil

1 cup red onion, thickly sliced

2 cups snap peas

¼ cup greek yogurt

2 tablespoons sriracha

Cooked ramen noodles for serving

Sesame seeds for serving

I HAVE tested these three different ways, and let me tell you, the air fryer is the way to go! If you do not have an air fryer, fear not! This dish is just as yummy baked in the oven or cooked solely in a cast-iron skillet on the stove top. Your options are endless, and one thing is for sure: this is going to be a delicious, hearty, family-favorite meal.

In a large bowl, mix the first ten ingredients, add 1 tablespoon of Sweet Chili Sauce, and work the mixture with your hands until fully combined. Scoop roughly 24 meatballs, roll between the palms of your hands, and place on a parchment-lined baking sheet. Freeze the meatballs for 20 minutes.

When ready to cook, set the air fryer temperature to 375°F/190°C. Place the meatballs into the basket in one layer, working in batches depending on the size of the basket. Cook the meatballs for 8–10 minutes or until the internal temperature reaches 165°F/73°C.

When the meatballs are nearly done, heat a large cast-iron skillet over medium-high heat. Add the olive oil to the pan. When the oil begins to shimmer, add the red onion and cook for 3–4 minutes until lightly charred. Add the snap peas and cook for an additional 2 minutes. Remove the cooked meatballs from the air fryer basket and add to the skillet with the onion and snap peas. Lastly, add the remaining 2 tablespoons of Sweet Chili Sauce and toss to coat. Remove the pan from the heat.

In a small bowl, stir the yogurt and sriracha together. Build your bowl: serve the meatballs over a bed of cooked ramen noodles, drizzle with the sriracha yogurt sauce, and top with scallions, cilantro, and sesame seeds.

SWEET CHILI SAUCE

YIELDS: 10 OUNCES
PREP TIME: 5 MINUTES
COOK TIME: 5–7 MINUTES

½ cup rice vinegar

½ cup water

½ cup plus 2 tablespoons granulated sugar

3 garlic cloves, grated

2 tablespoons sambal oelek

1 tablespoon rice wine (or 2 teaspoons mirin)

1 teaspoon fish sauce

1 teaspoon tamari

½ teaspoon dried Thai chilis, minced

4 teaspoons cornstarch

2 tablespoons water

Put the first nine ingredients into a small saucepan, and bring to a boil. Reduce the heat to low. In a small bowl, whisk the cornstarch and water to make a slurry. Slowly pour the slurry into the pot and stir continuously until thickened. Remove from the heat, cool slightly before pouring into a glass jar. Store in the refrigerator.

PINEAPPLE BBQ TURKEY MEAT LOAF

SERVES: 4
PREP TIME: 10 MINUTES
COOK TIME: 90 MINUTES

MEAT LOAF

½ cup panko

1 large egg plus 1 egg yolk

1 teaspoon worcestershire sauce

¼ cup Pineapple BBQ Glaze (see recipe below)

¼ cup sweet onion, grated

¼ cup green onion, diced

1½ pounds ground turkey

1 teaspoon salt

½ teaspoon pepper

Fresh-cut pineapple

Green onions, sliced for garnish

PINEAPPLE BBQ GLAZE

2 teaspoons olive oil

3 garlic cloves, minced

⅔ cup pineapple juice

½ cup teriyaki or island teriyaki sauce

½ cup ketchup

1 tablespoon maple syrup

1 teaspoon red pepper flakes

2 tablespoons freshly grated ginger

1 teaspoon cornstarch

1 tablespoon water

I AM often asked, "Did you get your love for cooking from your mom?" Truth be told, my memories recollect cooking to be the dredded chore after she'd worked, picked us up from school, and drove us to various sporting practices and after-school activities. This, however, is one of her specialties and shines with flavor creativity, proving she's a part of my love for cooking.

To start, prep the Pineapple BBQ Glaze. In a small saucepan, heat the olive oil over medium heat. Add the garlic, pineapple juice, teriyaki, ketchup, maple syrup, red pepper flakes, and fresh ginger. Bring to a simmer, then reduce heat to low and cook for about 25 minutes. Lastly, mix the cornstarch with water to make a slurry. Slowly stir the slurry into the sauce to thicken. Remove from the heat and set aside.

Preheat the oven to 325°F/160°C.

To make the meatloaf, add the panko, egg, egg yolk, worcestershire sauce, and ¼ cup of Pineapple BBQ Glaze to a large bowl. Whisk and let stand for 5 minutes. Add the onion, turkey, salt, and pepper. Mix with your hands until fully incorporated.

Transfer the meat mixture to an aluminum foil–lined baking sheet. Loosely form a meat loaf shape. Brush the meat loaf with ¼ cup of the glaze. Lay fresh pineapple around the loaf and bake for 60–75 minutes, until the internal temperature reaches 165°F/73°C.

Turn the broiler to high. Brush the meat loaf again with the glaze and broil for 3–5 minutes, being careful not to burn the top. Let the meat loaf rest for 5 minutes before serving. Serve each slice with roasted pineapple, green onions, and additional glaze to taste.

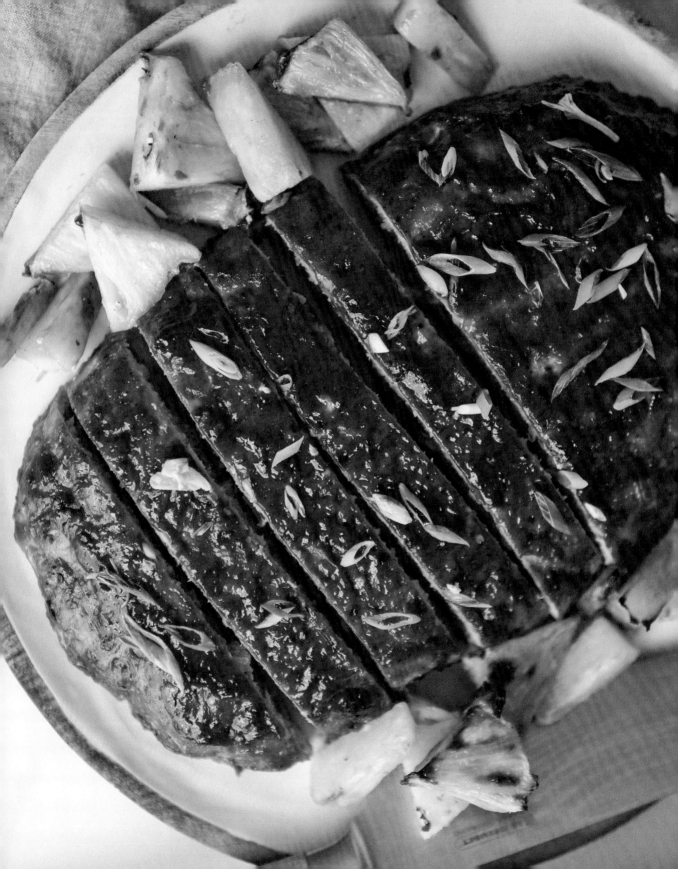

PORK CHOPS & BLUEBERRY-BALSAMIC JAM

SERVES: *4*
PREP TIME: *5 MINUTES*
COOK TIME: *35 MINUTES*

PORK CHOPS

4 boneless pork chops

Salt and pepper

2 tablespoons salted butter

2 bunches asparagus, woody ends trimmed

1 tablespoon olive oil

Kosher salt

1 teaspoon fresh thyme for serving

BLUEBERRY-BALSAMIC JAM

2 tablespoons honey

¼ cup balsamic vinegar

½ lemon, juiced

2 sprigs of fresh thyme

2 cups fresh (or frozen) blueberries

PORK CHOPS with the perfect layer of fat on the outer edge may be our absolute favorite cut of meat. Our shared earliest memories of pork chops are more associated with tough dry meat dunked in applesauce to help chew it down. We are rewriting those food memories and pumping up the flavor with each bite of this dish!

Preheat the oven to 425°F/220°C. Season the pork chops with salt and pepper to taste. Set aside while you prepare the Blueberry Balsamic Jam.

Combine the honey, balsamic vinegar, lemon juice, and sprigs of thyme in a small saucepan over medium heat. Bring to a low simmer for 2 minutes. Add the blueberries and cook until the berries are bursting, then reduce the heat to low and allow to thicken, about 5–7 minutes. Remove the pan from the heat and pick out the thyme sprigs, set aside.

To a large cast-iron skillet over medium heat, and the butter. Once the butter is melted, add the pork chops to sear. Cook for 3–4 minutes per side until golden brown.

Once the pork has been seared on all sides, move the cast-iron skillet to the hot oven. Cook in the oven until internal temperature reaches 145°F/63°C. Remove from the oven and sprinkle with fresh thyme.

Toss the trimmed asparagus on a baking sheet with olive oil and salt. Cook for 7–10 minutes while the pork is cooking.

Plate each pork chop with a dollop or two of the Blueberry-Balsamic Jam. Serve with a side of rice and roasted asparagus.

PRO TIP

Sear the fat-cap on the edge of the pork chops first to render the fat.

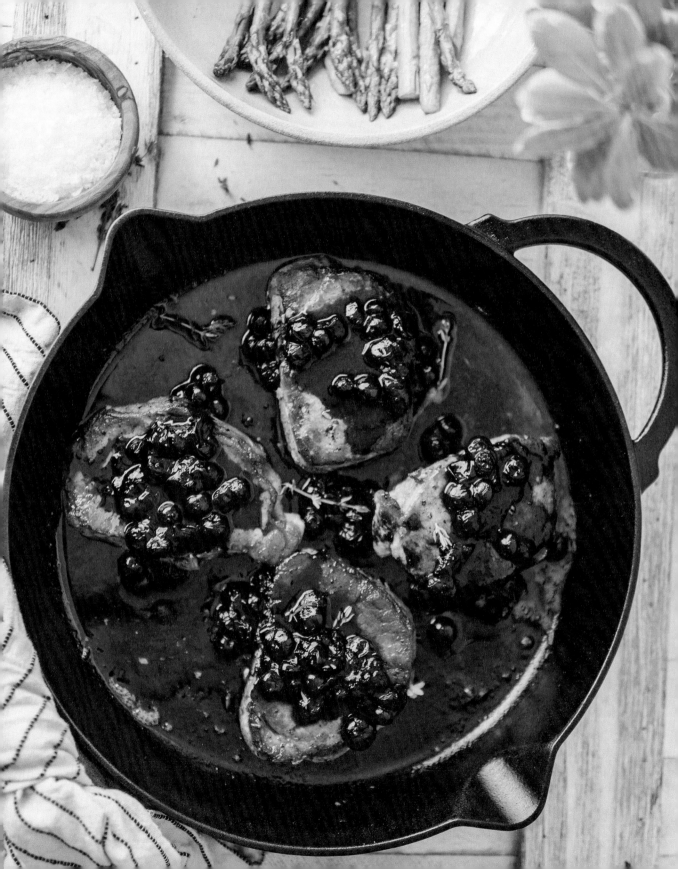

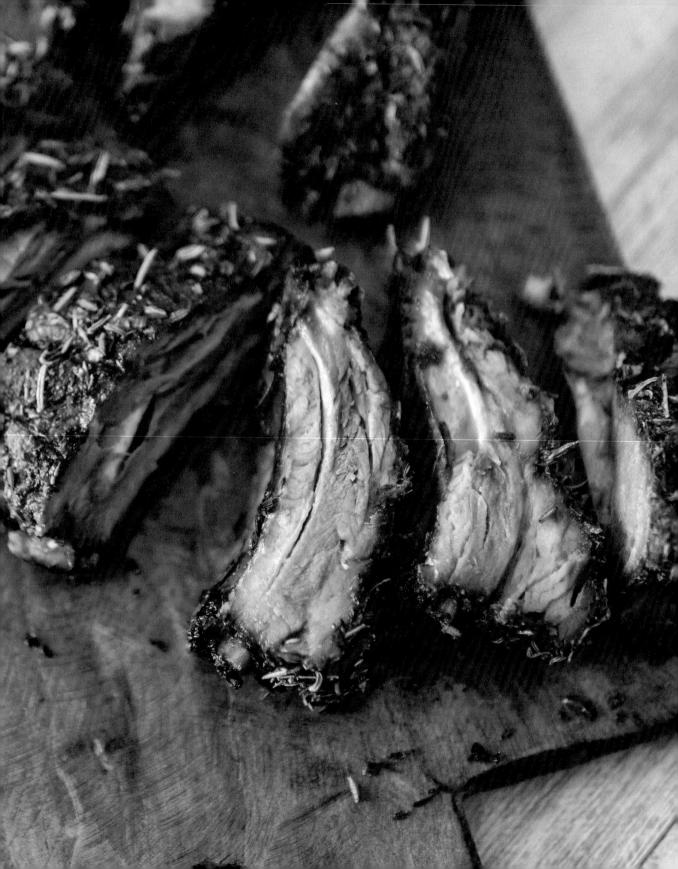

FENNEL RIBS

SERVES: 4–6
PREP TIME: 10 MINUTES
COOK TIME: 3½–4 HOURS

3 pounds pork ribs (baby back or St. Louis)

1½ tablespoons sea salt

2 tablespoons dijon mustard

1 tablespoon fennel seeds

1 tablespoon garlic powder

2 teaspoons thyme

2 teaspoons rosemary

1 teaspoon sage

¼ teaspoon dry mustard

ALL THESE bold, spiced ingredients stack up to a seriously complex bite. When these ribs are cooked to 204°F/95°C they fall right off the bone. After a few hours in the oven, your house will be filled with strong aromas and your mouth will be watering waiting for mealtime. Food is so strongly connected to our memories. These ribs remind me of summer days with our sweet Tennessee neighbors. That's where I learned how to cook these bold, herby ribs, and we haven't gone back to BBQ-sauced ribs since.

Prepare your ribs by removing any silver skin on the bone side if needed. Sprinkle with sea salt and slather with dijon mustard.

Using a mortar and pestle (bottom of a heavy fry pan or a rolling pin will work too!), slightly crush down the fennel seeds to help release the flavor. Place the crushed fennel into a small dish with the remaining spices. Season the ribs well with the mixture. Place the ribs in a large glass dish, cover with cling wrap, and refrigerate 4 hours up to overnight.

When ready to cook the ribs, remove from the fridge to allow them to come to room temperature while the oven preheats. Preheat the oven to 250°F/120°C.

Place the ribs on a baking sheet, bone-side down. Slow roast in the oven for 3½–4 hours or until internal temperature reaches 204°F/95°C. Remove the ribs from the oven, cover with aluminum foil, and rest for 10 minutes before slicing and serving.

SLOW COOKER CRISPY MOJO PORK BOWLS

SERVES: 6–8

PREP TIME: 15 MINUTES

COOK TIME: 4–6 HOURS OR 6–8 HOURS

¾ cup extra-virgin olive oil

¾ cup sour orange juice

½ cup fresh lime juice

1 cup cilantro leaves and stems

¼ cup fresh mint leaves

8 garlic cloves, smashed

1 tablespoon oregano

2 teaspoons ground cumin

1 teaspoon salt

1 teaspoon pepper

½ teaspoon red pepper flakes

3–5 pounds boneless pork butt

Jalapeño-Lime-Coconut White Rice (see page 140 for recipe) for serving

1 cup shredded swiss cheese for serving

Black beans for serving

Avocado, sliced for serving

Jalapeño, sliced for serving

ALL THE flavors of a classic Cuban sandwich served in a bowl. The combination of the citrus, cilantro, and mint with the crispy pork is the perfect marriage of flavors. I could stick a straw in the marinade and drink it down, it's that good!

Into the bowl of a food processor add olive oil, orange juice, lime juice, cilantro, mint, garlic, oregano, cumin, salt, pepper, and red pepper flakes. Blitz until smooth. Place the pork butt in a deep glass dish and pour the marinade over the pork to fully coat. Cover the dish and refrigerate for 4 hours up to overnight. When ready to cook, place the pork butt and marinade into the pot of a slow cooker. Cook on high for 4–6 hours or on low for 6–8 hours, until fork tender.

Remove the pork from the slow cooker and place on a baking sheet, reserving the cooking liquid. Preheat the broiler to high. While the oven preheats, shred the pork with 2 forks. Pour 1 cup of the reserved cooking liquid over the pork. Broil 5–7 minutes, checking frequently to ensure the pork is not burning, until browned and crispy.

Serve crispy pork over a bed of Jalapeño-Lime-Coconut White Rice with a sprinkle of swiss cheese, a scoop or two of black beans, and topped with slices of avocado and jalapeño.

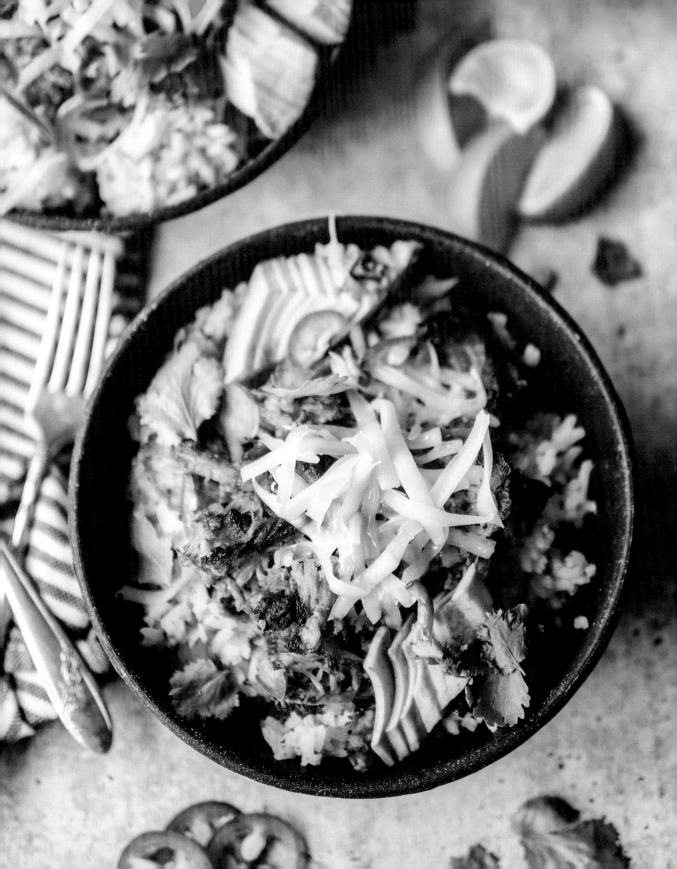

CHINESE BBQ PORK FRIED RICE

SERVES: 4

PREP TIME: 15 MINUTES (PLUS 2–24 HOURS MARINATING)

COOK TIME: 60 MINUTES

½ cup tamari (or soy sauce)

½ cup apricot preserves

¼ cup hoisin sauce

¼ cup white wine

¼ cup ketchup

2 tablespoons grated fresh ginger

1 tablespoon maple syrup

1 tablespoon toasted sesame oil

2 garlic cloves, grated

1 teaspoon pepper

½ teaspoon Chinese five-spice powder

3 tablespoons olive oil, divided

1 (2–2½ pounds) pork loin roast

4 cups cooked white rice

4 eggs, whites and yolks separated

8 ounces sugar snap peas, thinly sliced

8 ounces radish, halved and quartered

¼ cup green onion, minced

FRIED RICE is made at least once a week in our house. Like most meals I toss together, it's a great way to clean out the fridge of lingering veggies, rice, and prepared meats. You can even top it with a fried egg and serve it up for breakfast. When we're not winging it with leftovers, we're making a batch of this Chinese BBQ Pork Fried Rice and sharing each other's company over a warm, filling bowl.

In a large glass bowl, whisk the first eleven ingredients and 2 teaspoons of olive oil to make the marinade. Place the pork loin into the bowl, turning to fully coat. Cover and refrigerate for at least 2 hours up to overnight. When ready to cook, remove the pork from the fridge and let it sit on the counter for 30 minutes to remove the chill.

Preheat the oven to 375°F/190°C.

Heat a large cast-iron skillet over medium heat, add the remaining olive oil to the pan. When the oil shimmers, remove the pork from the marinade and place into the hot pan to sear, fat-side down first. Reserve the marinade for basting. Sear for 4-5 minutes on each side.

Move the cast-iron skillet to the preheated oven and roast for 10 minutes. At the 10-minute mark, flip the pork and brush with the reserved marinade. Roast for an additional 15–20 minutes. Baste with the reserved marinade 1–2 more times throughout the cook.

Remove the pork from the oven when the internal temperature reaches 140–145°F/60–62°C. Place the pork on a cutting board, cover with aluminum foil, and rest while you prepare the remaining ingredients. Save the cast-iron skillet with all the pork and marinade juices to cook the rice, place it on a burner over medium heat.

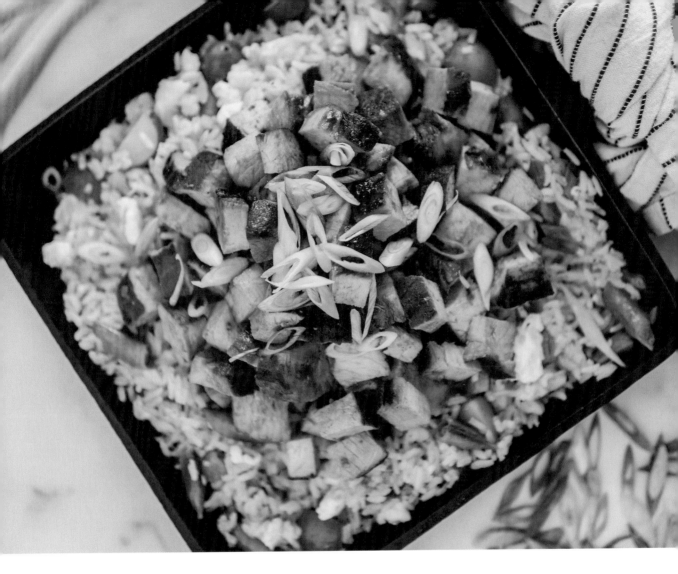

In a large bowl, working with your hands to fully incorporate, mix the cooked rice and the egg yolks. Add the rice to the skillet used to cook the pork and cook for 5 minutes. Move the rice to one side of the skillet, add the egg whites, and cook until scrambled. Once the eggs are cooked, mix them in with the rice. Add the sugar snap peas and radish to the skillet, toss to evenly incorporate. Spread the rice evenly over the skillet, cook an additional 3–5 minutes without touching to crisp the bottom of the rice.

While the rice finishes cooking, slice the pork. You can either serve the pork sliced on top of the rice or dice the pork into smaller pieces and mix in with the rice.

Just before serving, add the ¼ cup of green onion to the rice, toss, and serve immediately.

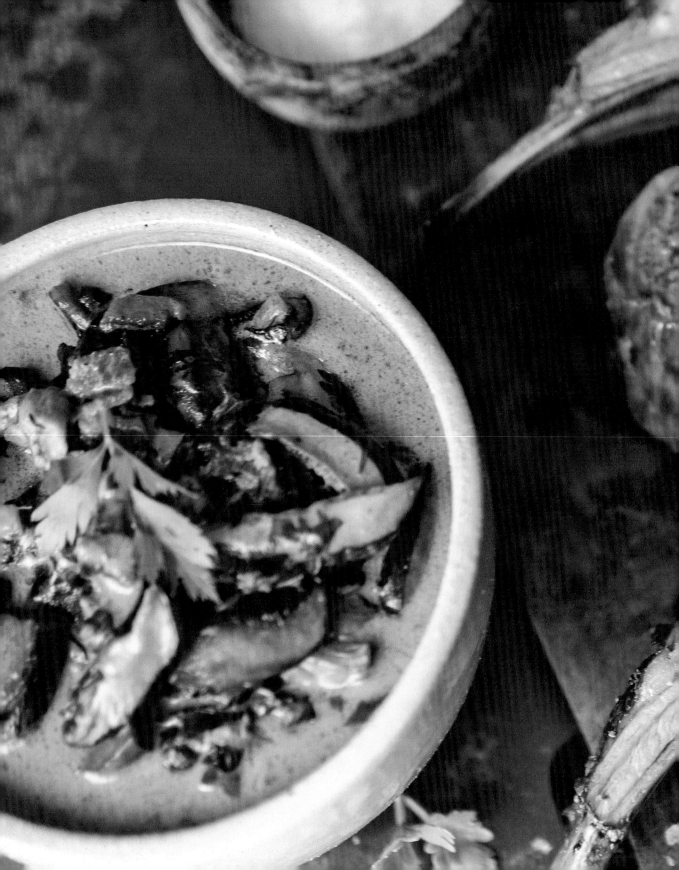

BEEF
& LAMB

SWEET CHILI ISLAND BISON BURGER

SERVES: 4–6
PREP TIME: 15 MINUTES
COOK TIME: 15 MINUTES

½ medium pineapple sliced into rounds, rind and core removed

2–4 tablespoons Sweet Chili Sauce (see page 77 for recipe)

1½ pounds ground bison

2 tablespoons tamari (or soy sauce)

2 tablespoons Pineapple BBQ Glaze (see page 78 for recipe)

Pinch cayenne pepper, salt, and pepper

6 slices swiss cheese

4–6 onion rolls

¼ cup mayo

8–12 slices fried bacon

Butter lettuce

MEET ME with a stash of napkins if there's a burger in my hands. I'm on Team "Don't Put It Down" once I've bitten into a burger. They're messy and delicious and meant to be enjoyed and savored. I don't want to be concerned about what's on my face while I'm taking in all the flavors of pineapple, BBQ, and bison. I'll wipe my face once it's gone!

Preheat the grill to 450–500°F/230–260°C.

Brush the pineapple rounds on each side with the Sweet Chili Sauce and set aside. In a large bowl, combine the ground bison, tamari, Pineapple BBQ Glaze, cayenne, salt, and pepper. Mix until combined and portion the mixture into 4–6 patties.

Grill the burgers and pineapple for 4–5 minutes, flip, and cook until the internal temperature reaches 130°F/55°C for medium rare and the pineapples are lightly charred and caramelized. During the last minute of grilling, add a slice of cheese to each patty.

While the cheese melts to the burgers, brush the inside of each onion roll with mayonnaise and place cut-side down on the grill.

When everything has finished cooking, remove the patties, pineapple, and buns from the grill and allow the patties to rest for 2 minutes. To assemble your burger, place two strips of bacon on the bottom buns. Top each with a burger patty, a slice of caramelized sweet chili pineapple, and a few leaves of butter lettuce. Add the top bun and enjoy!

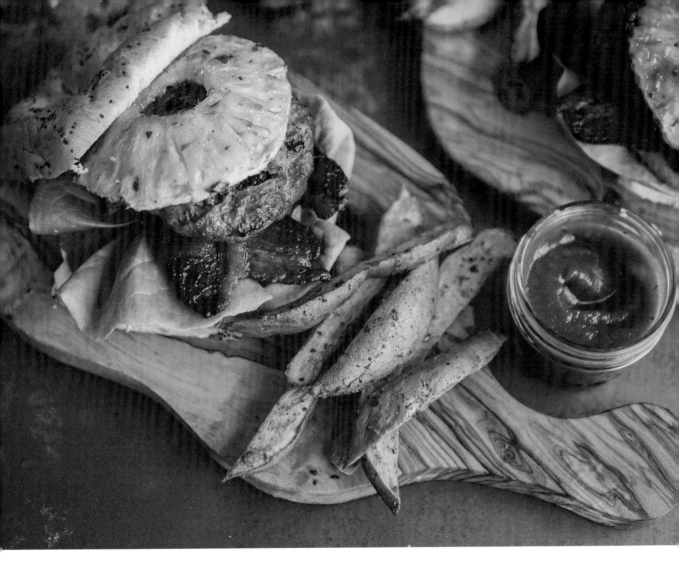

BEER-GLAZED ONION BURGER

SERVES: 4–6
PREP TIME: 15 MINUTES
COOK TIME: 45 MINUTES

2 tablespoons salted butter

3 sweet onions, thinly sliced

⅓ cup Mexican beer

1½ pounds ground beef

1 tablespoon worcestershire sauce

2 tablespoons dried minced onion

1 teaspoon onion powder

1 teaspoon dried parsley

½ teaspoon garlic powder

¼ teaspoon salt

4–6 slices provolone cheese

4–6 pretzel burger buns

4–6 tablespoons mayonnaise

Kettle-cooked chips for serving

BEER AND burgers on the grill, what's better than that? If you don't have a grill to fire up in the backyard, we also love smash burgers. You can cook your burgers on the stove top in a cast-iron skillet for an amazing crust and ultrathin patties. Get the pan searing hot, add a touch of olive oil, and press the burger patties flat with a spatula. Cook for 3–4 minutes, then flip!

In a large skillet over medium-low heat, add the butter. Once the butter is melted and slightly browned, add the sliced onions. Cook down, stirring occasionally for 15–20 minutes until golden brown. Add the beer and cook an additional 5–7 minutes until the alcohol has completely cooked off. Move to a plate, cover, and set aside until ready to serve.

While the onions cook, preheat the grill to 450–500°F/230–260°C.

In a medium bowl, combine the ground beef with the worcestershire sauce, dried minced onions, onion powder, garlic powder, dried parsley, and salt until fully combined. Portion the mixture into 4–6 patties.

Grill for 4–5 minutes, flip, and cook until the internal temperature reaches 130°F/55°C for medium rare. Remove the patties from the grill, top the burger with a heap of beer-glazed onions and a slice of provolone cheese. Let patties rest for 2 minutes to allow the cheese to melt into the burger.

Toast buns on the hot grill or in the oven under the broiler on high. Spread the mayonnaise on each burger bun. Place a burger patty on each of the bottom buns and close the bun. Serve with a side of kettle-cooked potato chips.

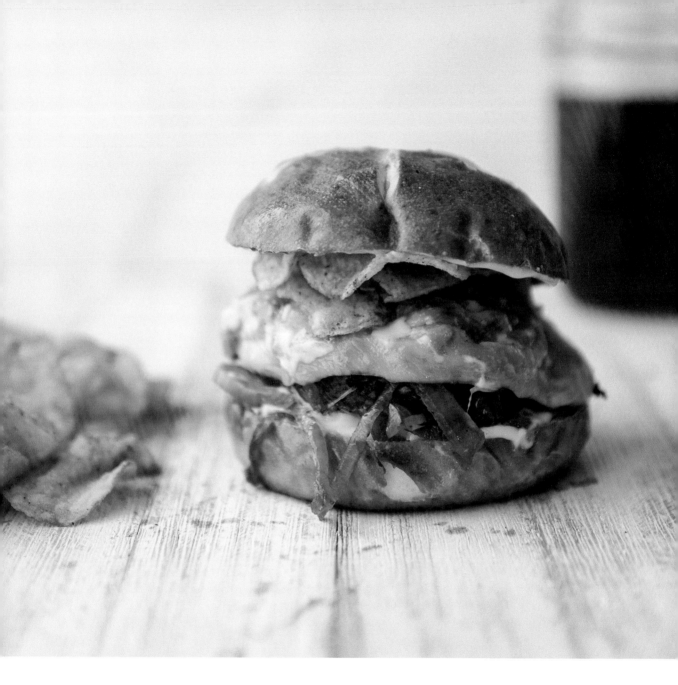

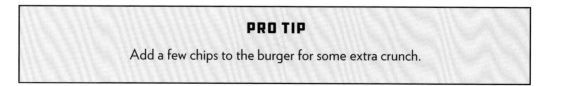

PRO TIP

Add a few chips to the burger for some extra crunch.

MOM'S AMERICAN CHOP SUEY

SERVES: 8
PREP TIME: 10 MINUTES
COOK TIME: 30 MINUTES

3 tablespoons olive oil

8 ounces cremini mushrooms, sliced

1 teaspoon kosher salt, divided

1 white onion, diced

2 teaspoons garlic, minced

1 green bell pepper, seeded and chopped

1 pound ground beef

½ teaspoon red pepper flakes

Black pepper to taste

2 (15-ounce) cans diced fire-roasted tomatoes, with juice

1 (15-ounce) can tomato sauce

1 (6-ounce) can tomato paste

⅔ cup beef broth

¼ cup fresh basil, chopped (plus more for garnish)

1 teaspoon fresh oregano

1 teaspoon worcestershire sauce

1 tablespoon granulated sugar

1 pound elbow macaroni

8 ounces ricotta

4–6 English muffins

4 tablespoons salted butter

4 tablespoons basil pesto

Freshly grated Parmesan

ANOTHER CHILDHOOD favorite and a dish that was always on the buffet table at a potluck. My mom would make a big batch of this, knowing it stores and reheats well. A hungry kid in our house lingering by an open fridge door in search of something to eat was likely to find this on the bottom shelf waiting for them.

Heat olive oil in a large skillet over medium heat. When the oil shimmers, add the mushrooms and a ½ teaspoon of salt. Cook for 5 minutes until browned. Add the onions, garlic and green peppers, cook for 3-5 minutes. To the skillet add the ground beef, breaking up into small pieces. Cook for 5-7 minutes until no pink remains. Add the red pepper flakes, remaining salt, and pepper. Lastly, add the tomatoes, tomato sauce, tomato paste, beef broth, basil, oregano, worcestershire sauce, and granulated sugar. Simmer for 5 minutes.

While the meat sauce is simmering, cook the pasta to package instructions. When the pasta is done, strain from the water but do not rinse. Add the pasta and meat sauce to a large 9x13 baking dish for serving, toss to fully incorporate.

Add the ricotta to a food processor and whip for 2–3 minutes until smooth.

Preheat the broiler to high. Lay the English muffins cut-side up on a baking sheet. In a small bowl, mix the butter and basil pesto. Butter each English muffin generously with the pesto butter, and broil for 3–5 minutes until golden.

Scoop a hearty portion of pasta topped with a dollop of whipped ricotta and grated Parmesan. Serve each dish with the English Muffin Garlic Bread on the side.

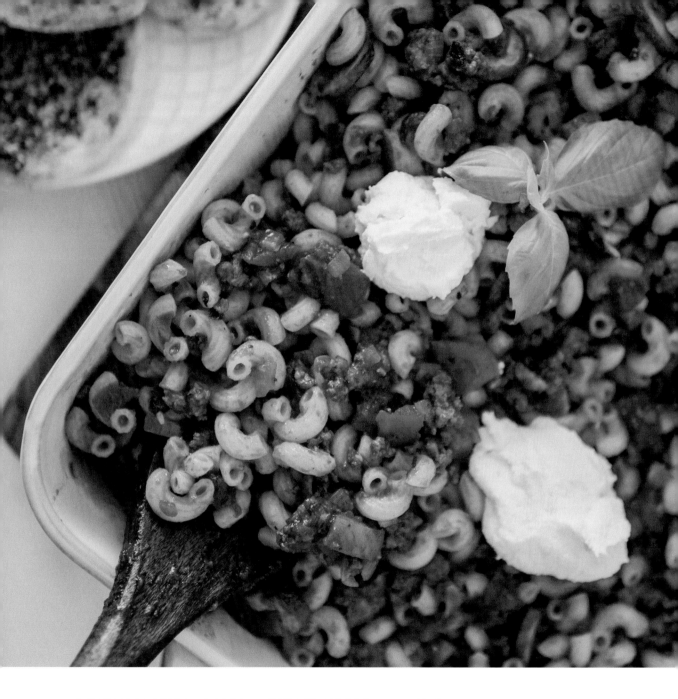

PRO TIP

You *can* skip whipping the ricotta, but it takes out the graininess of the ricotta and makes it extra creamy.

REVERSE-SEARED STEAK WITH BALSAMIC-ROASTED GRAPES & DIJON CABBAGE

SERVES: 4
PREP TIME: 15 MINUTES
COOK TIME: 50 MINUTES

1 tablespoon salt, plus more to taste

1 tablespoon pepper, plus more to taste

1 tablespoon garlic powder

4 2-inch thick rib eye steaks

2 cups red grapes

3–4 sprigs fresh thyme

2 tablespoons balsamic vinegar, divided

½ cup olive oil, divided

½ green cabbage, cut into 2-inch slices

½ red cabbage, cut into 2-inch slices

1 tablespoon whole-grain dijon mustard

½ teaspoon red pepper flakes

THIS IS a great meal for entertaining. Once you've got the components together, toss them all in the oven and smoker, and get ready to impress. I've made these steaks both in the oven and on the smoker. For this recipe, we are going to utilize the smoker to free up the space in the oven for our sides. **If you do not have a smoker and you're using a conventional grill, only turn half the burners on and place the steaks on the cool side of the grill during the low-heat cooking step.

Preheat the oven to 400°F/200°C, and preheat the smoker/grill to 200°F/95°C.

In a small bowl, mix the salt, pepper, and garlic powder. Season steaks generously with this mix. Set aside.

On a small, rimmed baking sheet, toss the grapes with the sprigs of thyme, 1 tablespoon of balsamic vinegar, 2 tablespoons of olive oil, and a pinch of salt. Cover the tray with aluminum foil and set aside.

On a separate large, rimmed baking sheet, lay the sliced cabbage, leaving a bit of space between. Drizzle with 2 tablespoons of olive oil and sprinkle with a pinch or two of salt. Flip and work the olive oil in with your hands to fully coat.

Once the oven and smoker have come to temperature, place the cabbage into the oven and the steaks directly on the grates.** Set the timer for 20 minutes. At 20 minutes, flip the cabbage and return to the oven. Add the tray of grapes to the oven. Roast the grapes and cabbage for an additional 20 minutes.

When the steaks have been slow-cooked for 30–40 minutes, and the internal temperature is around

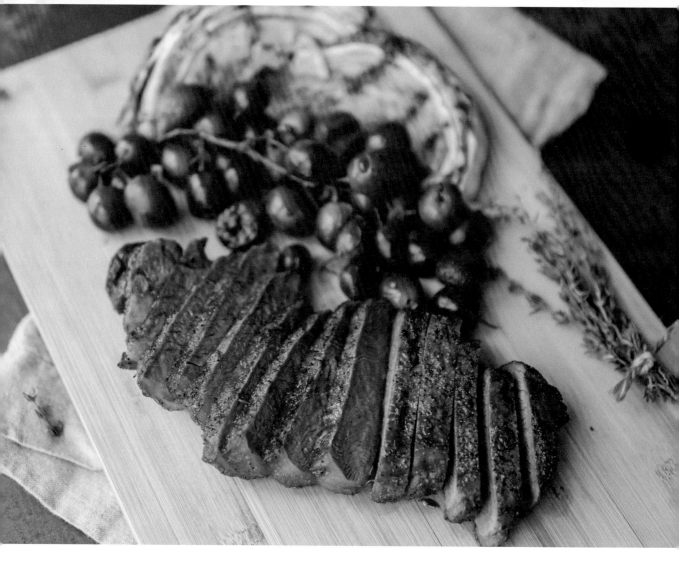

120°F/48°C, remove the steaks from the smoker and increase the temperature to 450–500°F/230–260°C. Sear the steaks for 2–3 minutes on each side and remove when the internal temperature reaches 135°F/57°C for medium rare. Rest for 5–7 minutes before slicing.

In a small bowl, whisk the remaining ¼ cup of olive oil, dijon, the remaining 1 tablespoon of balsamic vinegar, red pepper flakes, salt, and pepper. Drizzle the dressing over the roasted cabbage just before serving.

Serve each steak with a side of roasted cabbage topped with the balsamic roasted grapes.

** The steaks can be done low and slow in the oven at 200°F/95°C and then seared on a conventional grill or stove top in a cast-iron skillet. You will not get that wood-fired smoky flavor, but the method remains the same!

BEEF & LAMB

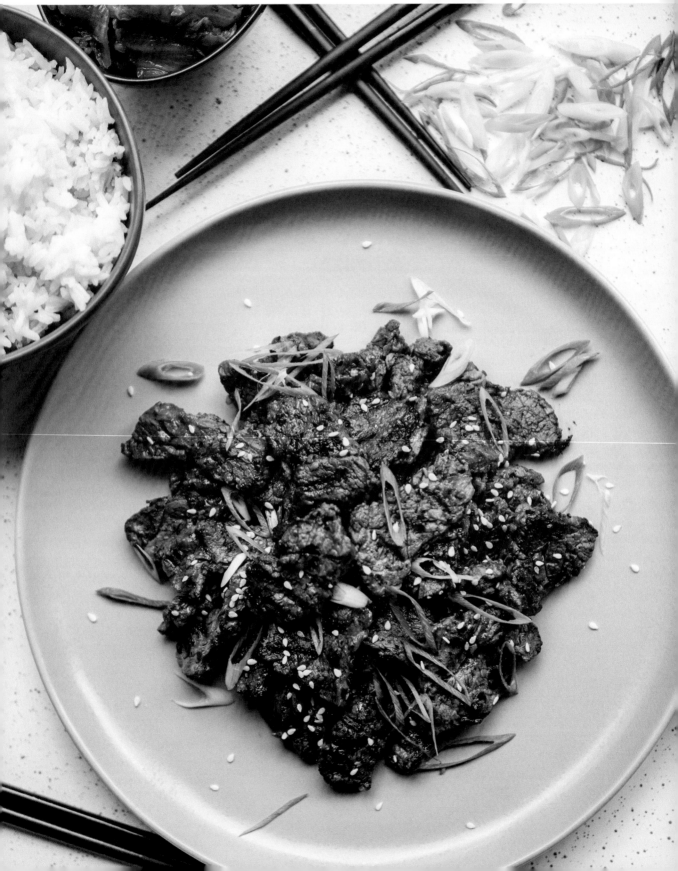

BEEF BULGOGI

SERVES: 4
PREP TIME: 10 MINUTES (PLUS
2–4 HOURS MARINATING)
COOK TIME: 20 MINUTES

3 tablespoons tamari (or soy sauce)

2 tablespoons red wine

2 tablespoons minced garlic

1 tablespoon toasted sesame oil

½ teaspoon ground black pepper

1 teaspoon red pepper flakes

1 kiwi, finely chopped

4 green onions, sliced thin and divided

1 pound trimmed flank steak, sliced thin

2 tablespoons olive oil

2 teaspoons toasted sesame seeds for serving

2 cups steamed white rice for serving

½ cup kimchi for serving

BULGOGI IS most often made with rib eye steaks and cooked over a live fire. In this recipe, the winning ingredient is the kiwi! Believe it or not, kiwi acts as a tenderizer for the beef. It adds a hint of natural sweetness to the marinade but mainly helps break down the surface proteins and enhances the flavor of the beef. These chargrilled pieces of steak melt in your mouth!

In a large bowl, whisk the tamari, red wine, minced garlic, toasted sesame oil, black pepper, red pepper flakes, kiwi, and 2 tablespoons of sliced green onions. Add the sliced flank steak to the bowl. Toss to fully coat in the marinade. Cover and chill in the refrigerator for at least 2 hours. (Do not exceed 4 hours, as the kiwi will break down the meat too much and you will end up with mushy steak.)

After 2 hours, remove the steak from the fridge and allow it to sit on the counter for 30 minutes.

Heat a cast-iron skillet over high heat. Pour 1 tablespoon of olive oil into the skillet. When the oil shimmers, add ½ the beef to the hot pan in one layer, allowing space between the pieces to help crisping. Cook for 1–2 minutes on each side and then move to a separate clean plate. Repeat this process with the remaining steak; heat oil and cook the steak for 1–2 minutes on each side until lightly browned.

Sprinkle the lightly charred steak with toasted sesame seeds and the remaining sliced green onions. Serve immediately with a side of steamed white rice and kimchi.

SHREDDED PORTUGUESE BEEF BOWLS

SERVES: 6–8

PREP TIME: 20 MINUTES (PLUS 4–24 HOURS MARINATING)

COOK TIME: 3½ HOURS

2½ pounds chuck roast, cubed

½ cup crushed red peppers (this is a wet ingredient found in most international food aisles, not dry red pepper flakes)

1 large onion, halved and quartered

8 garlic cloves, peeled and smashed

2 bay leaves

⅛ teaspoon nutmeg

⅛ teaspoon ground cloves

½ teaspoon ground cinnamon

2 tablespoons tomato paste

2 cups red wine

3 tablespoons salted butter, cubed

2 pounds baby Yukon Gold potatoes, quartered

2 tablespoons olive oil

2 teaspoons oregano

1 teaspoon red pepper flakes

2 teaspoons flaky salt

2 cups cooked white rice

Hot pepper rings, diced for serving

THIS IS a recipe that reminds me of my childhood, growing up in a predominantly Portuguese corner of the world. The inspiration for this meal is called caçoila (pronounced ka-SIR-la) and is traditionally cooked with pork butt/shoulder, served on a soft, flour-dusted Portuguese roll. This recipe brings all the flavors of childhood memories together in one bowl.

In a large bowl, toss the cubed chuck roast with the crushed red peppers. Cover and refrigerate for 4 hours up to overnight.

When ready to cook, place the onions, garlic, and bay leaves into a dutch oven or heavy-bottomed pot. Add the chuck roast. In a medium bowl, whisk the nutmeg, ground cloves, cinnamon, tomato paste, and wine. Pour over the roast. Top with the cubes of butter.

Bring the pot to a boil, reduce the heat to a simmer, cover, and cook for 1½–2 hours on low. Remove the cover and continue to cook on low for an additional 1–1½ hours.

In the last half of the meat cooking, prepare the potatoes. Preheat the oven to 400°F/200°C. In a large bowl, toss the potatoes with olive oil, oregano, red pepper flakes, and salt to evenly coat. Using two baking sheets, spread the potatoes in one layer with plenty of space to allow crisping. Roast the potatoes for 15–20 minutes, toss and return to the oven for another 15–20 minutes until golden.

When the meat is fork tender, shred the beef in the pot and assemble the bowl for serving. Lay down cooked white rice, spoon a heaping serving of beef and sauce over the rice. Add a side of crispy potatoes and top with diced hot pepper rings.

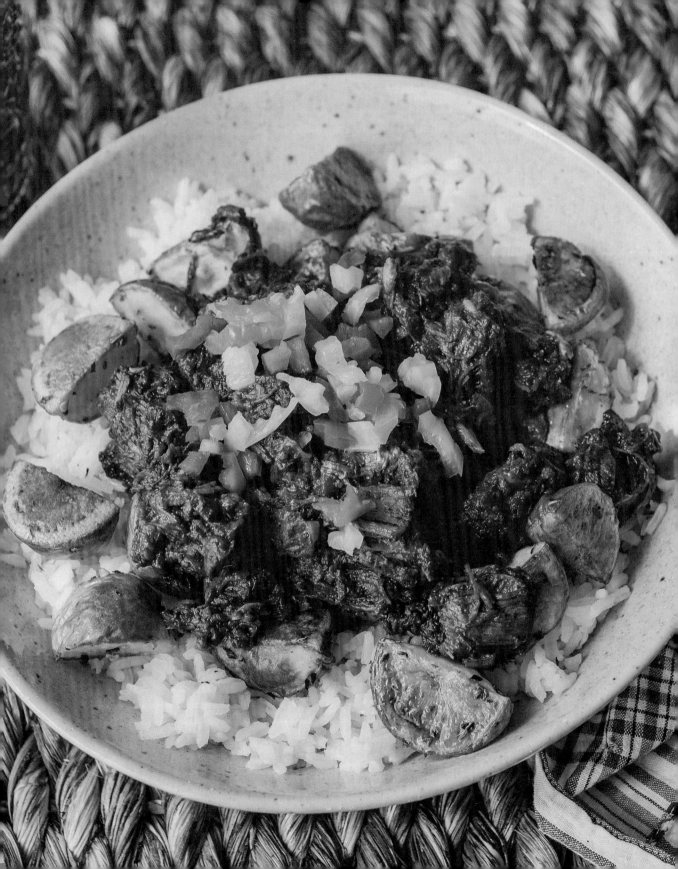

PEPPERONCINI BEEF CHILI

SERVES: *4–6*
PREP TIME: *10 MINUTES*
COOK TIME: *6–8 HOURS***

3 pounds chuck roast, cubed

1 tablespoon salt

1 tablespoon olive oil

1 small sweet onion, diced

3 cloves garlic, minced

1 tablespoon chili powder

2 tablespoons dried oregano

2 teaspoons smoked paprika

2 teaspoons cumin

1 teaspoon dried thyme

½ teaspoon red pepper flakes

1 dried bay leaf

1 (14-ounce) jar fire-roasted tomatoes

6 ounces tomato paste

10 ounces canned beef consommé

1 (16-ounce) jar pepperoncini plus liquid

½ cup balsamic vinegar

15 ounces great northern beans, drained and rinsed

¼ cup sun-dried tomatoes in olive oil, roughly chopped

1 bunch escarole, chopped

5 ounces grated Parmesan cheese

½ cup chopped parsley

THIS IS the love child of chili and Italian beef. I'm a sucker for a warm, saucy bowl of stewed ingredients just begging for crusty bread to dip into it. This is comfort and warmth in a bowl. I think I subconsciously make recipes like this when I'm going to be out of the house for the day just so I can come home and be hit with the warm smell of dinner when I walk in the door. Is there anything better?

Toss the cubes of chuck roast with salt to season. Heat the tablespoon of olive oil in a large cast-iron skillet over medium-high heat. When the oil shimmers, add the beef in two batches. Sear on each side for about 5 minutes or until a nice dark crust forms. While the beef sears, mix all ingredients from onion to sun-dried tomatoes into the pot of a 6-quart slow cooker. The escarole, Parmesan, and parsley will be added just before serving. Whisk to combine, and add the beef as it finishes searing. Once all the beef is added, cover and cook on low for 6–8 hours or on high for 4–6 hours. About 15 minutes before serving, add the chopped escarole. Stir to combine. Remove the large chunks of beef and slightly shred, either on a cutting board or right in the pot. Finish the chili by adding the Parmesan and parsley. Serve with a large cut of crusty bread spread with salted butter for dipping.

** 4–6 hours on high / pressure cooker: 90 Minutes

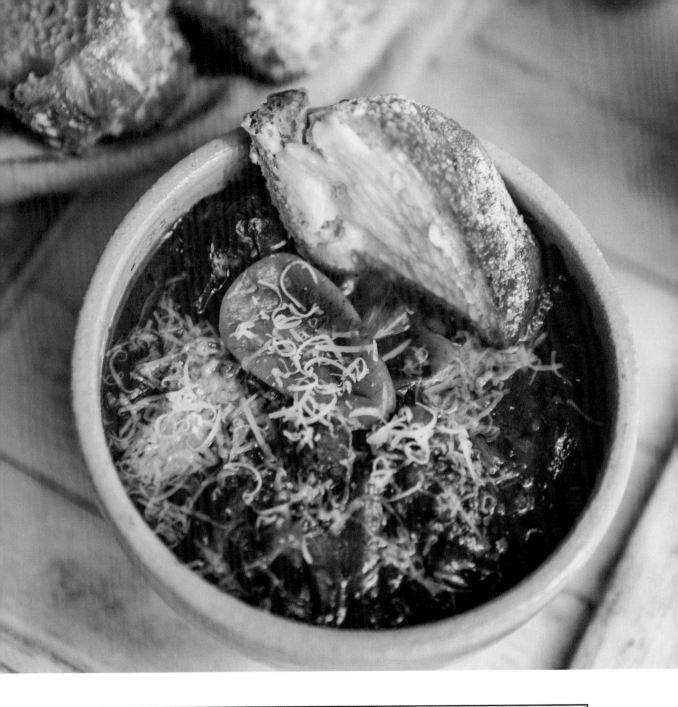

PRO TIP

Lay the beef in the hot pan with a bit of space between each piece. Do not push the beef around; this will help form a crust.

ROASTED RACK OF LAMB WITH COCONUT-BACON GRAVY

LAMB

2 racks of lamb

Salt and pepper to taste

1 tablespoon garlic, grated

1 tablespoon dijon mustard

1 teaspoon oregano

COCONUT-BACON GRAVY

4 slices thick-cut bacon

1 pint cremini mushrooms, sliced

2 pints shiitake mushrooms, sliced

¼ cup onion, diced

2 tablespoons shallots, minced

2 (15-ounce) cans full-fat coconut milk

½ cup cilantro leaves

½ cup parsley leaves, plus more for garnish

½ teaspoon cayenne pepper

Fresh cracked black pepper to taste

Kosher salt to taste

Steamed white rice

Steamed broccoli

I'M PRETTY sure this is one of Mat's favorite meals, ever. Like many meals we re-create at home, we originally had this meal while traveling abroad. While on a work trip in Belgium, we were invited to have dinner with a sweet family in town. Dinner was a simple spinach salad, lamb, and a thick coconut gravy. We could not get enough of the gravy, filled with dices of bacon and meaty cuts of mushroom. I got back to our hotel and wrote down a list of everything I tasted to be able to come home and re-create it.

On a baking sheet, season lamb generously with salt and pepper to taste. Rub the lamb with the grated garlic, dijon, and oregano. Refrigerate at least 2–4 hours to marinate.

While the lamb is marinating, prepare the Coconut-Bacon Gravy.

Preheat the oven to 350°F/177°C. Lay the strips of bacon on an aluminum foil-lined baking sheet. Bake the bacon for 15–20 minutes or until desired doneness. (We prefer slightly crisp.) Remove the bacon from the oven, reserving 2 tablespoons of bacon grease. Lay the bacon on a paper towel–lined plate. Once cooled, chop the bacon and set aside.

In a saucepan, heat the bacon grease over medium heat. Add the mushrooms to cook down and brown, about 7–10 minutes. Add the diced onions and shallots. Cook for about 5 minutes until translucent and slightly browned, adding a pinch of salt. Next, add the chopped bacon. Pour the cans of coconut milk into the pot. Reduce heat to a simmer and cook, stirring occasionally for 30 minutes until slightly reduced. Add the cilantro, parsley, and cayenne pepper and a pinch or two of fresh

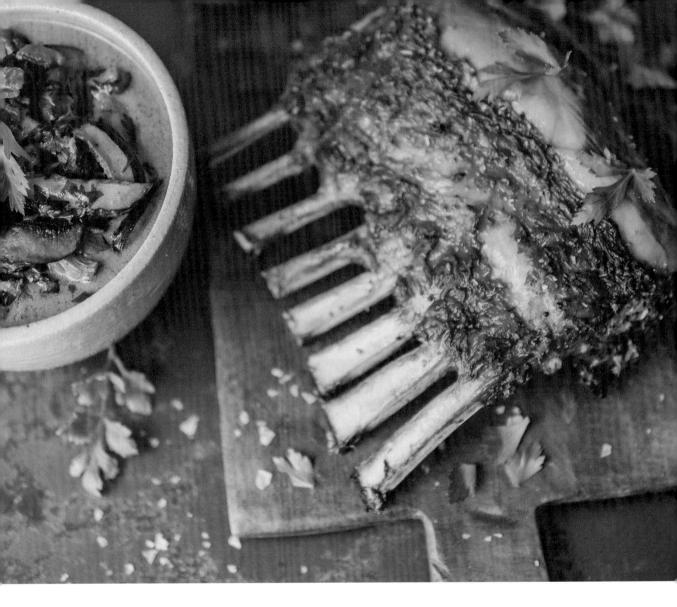

cracked black pepper to taste. Continue to cook uncovered for an additional 30 minutes on low heat. The gravy should be reduced and slightly thickened. Taste and adjust salt as needed.

Rest the lamb on the counter while the oven preheats. Preheat the oven to 450°F/230°C. Lay the rack of lamb on a rimmed baking sheet, bone-side down.

Roast for 10 minutes. Reduce the oven temperature to 300°F/150°C and roast an additional 15–20 minutes or until the internal temperature reaches 125°F/51°C. Remove the lamb from the oven and rest for 10 minutes before slicing. Cut into the rack at every two bones for serving. Serve each cut over steamed white rice, smothered in Coconut-Bacon Gravy along with a side of steamed broccoli.

BEEF & LAMB

LAMB KABOBS WITH HARISSA HONEY CARROTS & CHICKPEAS

SERVES: 4–6

PREP TIME: 15 MINUTES (PLUS 4–24 HOURS MARINATING)

COOK TIME: 40 MINUTES

MARINADE

½ cup dry white wine

½ cup olive oil

3 tablespoons lemon juice

8 garlic cloves, minced

4 teaspoons salt

4 teaspoons honey

4 teaspoons whole-grain mustard

1 tablespoon fresh oregano, chopped

2 teaspoons red pepper flakes

Pinch black pepper

LAMB AND CARROTS

2 pounds trimmed leg of lamb, cut into 1-inch cubes

2 pounds rainbow carrots, peeled

¼ cup olive oil, divided

2 teaspoons cumin, divided

2 tablespoons honey

2 tablespoons harissa sauce

Salt and pepper to taste

1 (15-ounce) can chickpeas, drained and patted dry

1 cup plain greek yogurt

THERE IS a LOT of flavor in this dish. The laundry list of ingredients may seem daunting, but I promise you, it's actually a very simple recipe. It was so hard to pull back because each ingredient helps bring so much flavor to the meat or to the veggies, each deserve their spot on the list! Harissa is a North African blend of hot peppers, oils, and spices. It can be found in many grocery stores.

In a large bowl, whisk all the marinade ingredients. Add the cubed lamb, toss to evenly coat, and push the lamb into the marinade to submerge. Cover and chill in the fridge for 4 hours or, ideally, overnight.

Preheat the oven to 425°F/220°C.

On a large baking sheet, combine the carrots, 2 tablespoons of olive oil, 1 teaspoon of cumin, honey, harissa, and salt and pepper to taste. Toss well to evenly coat. Place in the oven and roast for 15 minutes. Remove from the oven, add the chickpeas and the remaining olive oil to the sheet. Toss with the carrots and return to the oven to roast for an additional 20 minutes or until the chickpeas are crisp and the carrots are tender and lightly browned.

In a small bowl, mix yogurt and remaining cumin. Chill in the fridge until ready to serve.

When ready to cook the lamb, preheat the grill to 450°F/230°C. Distribute the cubes of lamb evenly onto skewers. Grill, flipping once or twice to evenly char and until the internal temperature reaches 125°F/51°C, about 10–15 minutes. Remove the skewers from the grill and rest for 10 minutes before serving.

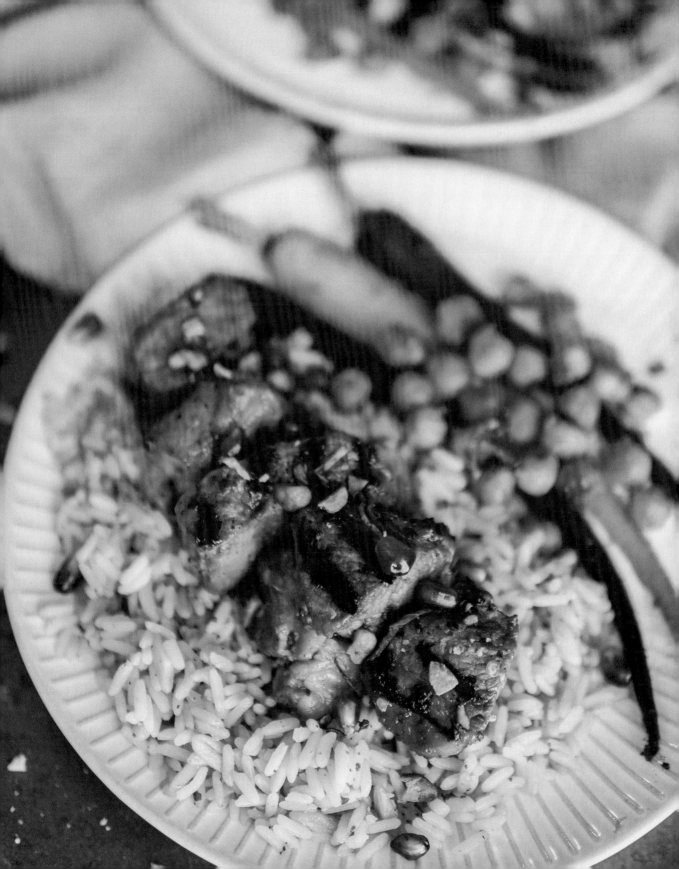

Cooked rice pilaf for serving

Mint leaves, pomegranate seeds, feta cheese, and crushed pistachios, for garnish

To assemble, evenly distribute the yogurt on the bottom of the plates. Top with honey harissa carrots and crispy chickpeas and lamb skewers. Garnish each plate with mint leaves, pomegranate seeds, crumbled feta, and crushed pistachios.

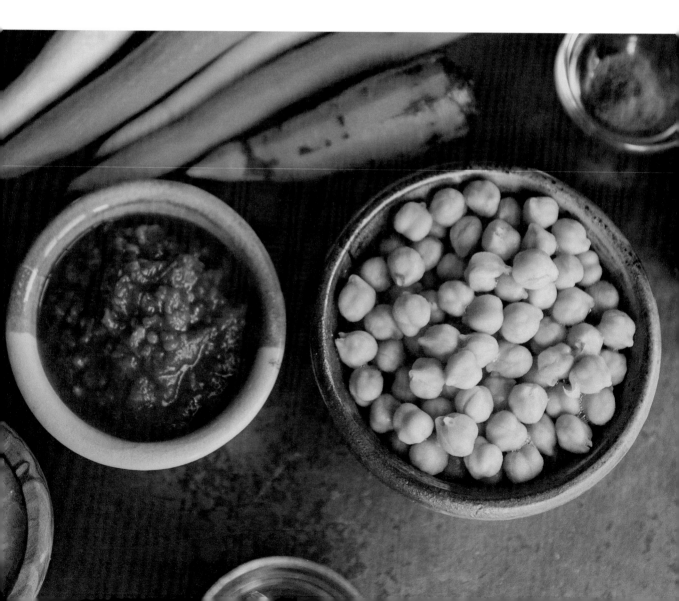

THAI BEEF BASIL WITH CRISPY SHALLOTS

SERVES 4
PREP TIME: 10 MINUTES
COOK TIME: 25 MINUTES

1 tablespoon plus 2 teaspoons tamari (or soy sauce)

2 teaspoons maple syrup

2 teaspoons oyster sauce

1 teaspoon hoisin sauce

2 tablespoons fish sauce

½ teaspoon red pepper flakes

2 tablespoons olive oil, divided

1 pound ground beef

Kosher salt to taste

2 pints shiitake mushrooms, sliced

½ cup sweet onion, thinly sliced

1 red bell pepper, sliced

5 cloves garlic, thinly sliced

1 cup sweet basil

½ cup mint leaves

8 ounces angel hair vermicelli noodles (cooked to package instructions)

Serrano peppers, sliced for serving

Crispy Shallots for serving (see recipe on page 111)

IT'S NOT often we order takeout these days, but we both have childhood memories of local dining spots our families would frequent on special occasions. For both of us, we remember take-out containers of General Tso's and pad thai. I'm excited to learn about unique and new flavors to share with my family and friends and bring food experiences home.

In a small bowl, mix the tamari, maple syrup, oyster sauce, hoisin sauce, fish sauce, and red pepper flakes. Set aside.

In a large cast-iron skillet (or wok if you have one!), heat half the olive oil over medium heat. When the oil shimmers, add the ground beef. Break it up from its packaged puck to spread it out. Resist the urge to push it around; this will help create a crust and texture in the beef. Cook until little pink remains, about 5–7 minutes, and then begin to break it up into small pieces. Season with salt and cook for an additional minute. Move the beef to a plate and set aside.

Add the remaining half of the olive oil to the same skillet over medium heat. Add the shiitake mushrooms, cook for 5–7 minutes or until browned. Turn the heat up to high and add the onion and red bell pepper. Cook for 2–3 minutes until lightly charred. Lastly, add the garlic and cook, stirring often for 2 minutes. Return the beef to the skillet along with the sauce ingredients. Toss to combine. Reduce the heat to medium-low and cook 1–2 minutes until the sauce is fully incorporated. Turn the heat off. Add the basil and mint, toss to incorporate.

Serve the beef over the cooked vermicelli noodles, garnished with serrano peppers and Crispy Shallots.

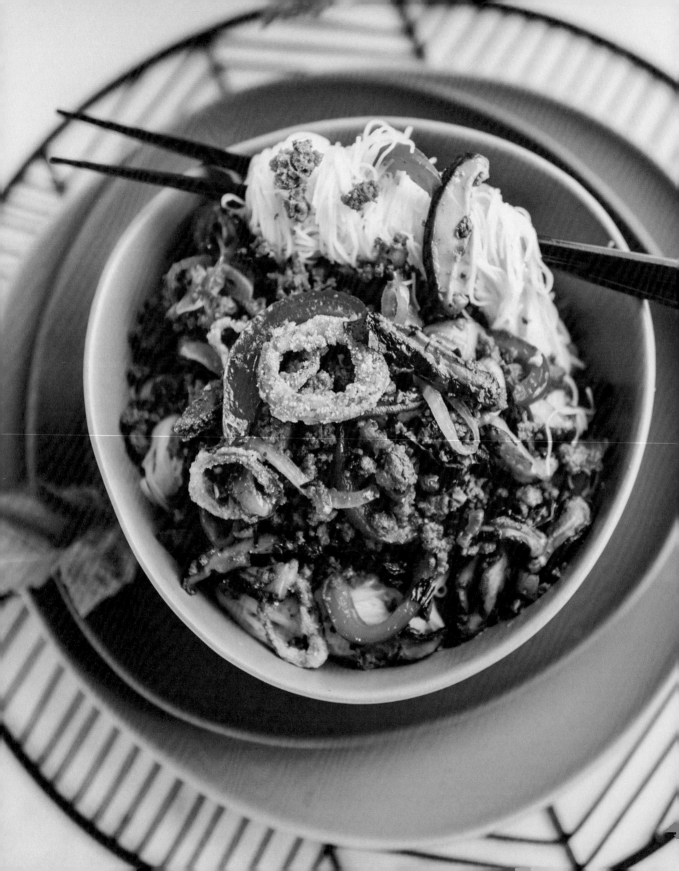

CRISPY SHALLOTS

YIELDS: ¼ CUP
PREP TIME: 15-20 MINUTES
COOK TIME: 8-10 MINUTES

1 shallot, thinly sliced

¼ cup buttermilk (whole milk will also work just fine)

1 tablespoon olive oil

½ cup white cornmeal

STORE-BOUGHT IS an alternative here, but these crispy shallots are easy to prepare while the beef is cooking in the cast-iron skillet. Best used immediately. They add a nice texture to the dish and a pop of flavor.

Before you prep your dinner ingredients, get the shallots into a small bowl with the buttermilk to rest for 15-20 minutes. While the beef is cooking on the stove top, heat a small skillet over medium-high heat with the olive oil.

Place the cornmeal into a shallow dish. Using a fork, or your fingers, strain the shallots from the milk, shaking off any excess liquid. Dredge the shallots through the cornmeal, shaking off any excess before laying into the hot oil.

Working in two batches, fry the shallots for 1–2 minutes on each side or until golden. Remove from the oil and place on a paper towel–lined plate. Serve immediately on top of the Thai Beef Basil dish.

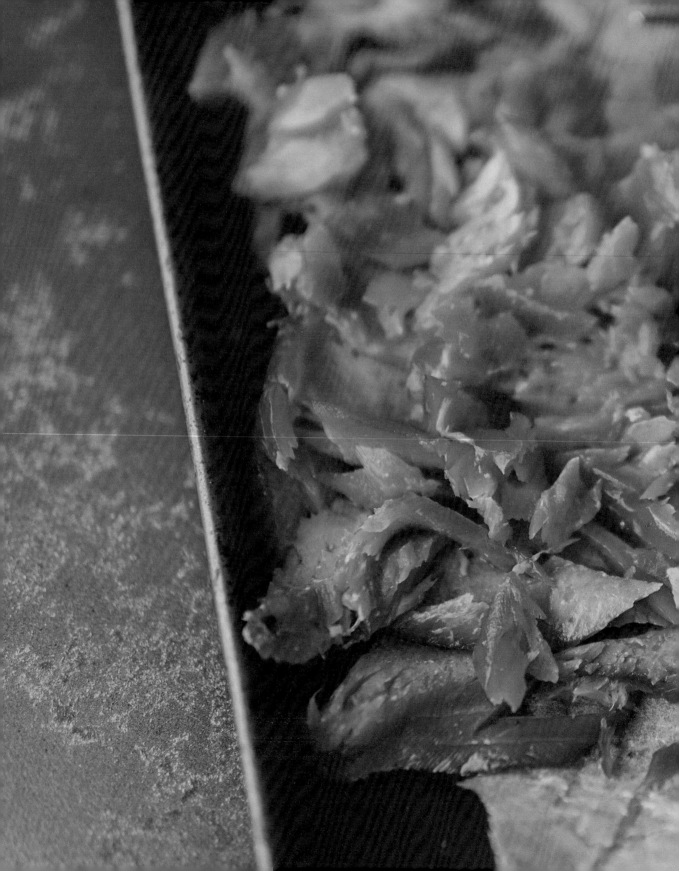

SEAFOOD

BLACKENED MAHI MAHI & JALAPEÑO-MINT-MANGO SALSA

SERVES: 4
PREP TIME: 15 MINUTES
COOK TIME: 15 MINUTES

2 teaspoons smoked paprika

2 teaspoons salt

2 teaspoons black pepper

1 teaspoon garlic salt

1 teaspoon dried parsley

1 teaspoon dried minced onion

1 teaspoon cayenne pepper

1 teaspoon oregano

2 tablespoons olive oil, divided

4 (4-ounce) mahi mahi fillets

Lime wedges for serving

2 cups cooked white rice (or Jalapeño-Lime-Coconut White Rice on page 140)

Jalapeño-Mint-Mango Salsa (see page 181 for recipe)

IF YOU are new to eating and cooking fish, mahi mahi is a great entry into seafood. Mahi mahi is sweet and has a very mild fish flavor. It's much leaner than say, salmon, and its meat is tender. It's pretty much a blank canvas just waiting for flavors to absorb. A fish like this holds up to strong spices and sweet and spicy salsa like the Jalapeño-Mint-Mango Salsa.

In a small bowl, mix the first eight ingredients for the blackening seasoning. Pour 1 tablespoon of olive oil over mahi mahi, and gently rub evenly into each piece of fish. Generously season the oiled fish with blackening seasoning.

Heat a large cast-iron skillet over medium heat with the remaining tablespoon of olive oil. When the oil shimmers, add the mahi mahi. Cook for 5–7 minutes before flipping. Cook an additional 3–4 minutes or until the internal temperature reads 145°F/62°C. Remove from the cast-iron skillet. Squeeze lime wedge over fish.

Serve mahi mahi topped with Jalapeño-Mint-Mango Salsa.

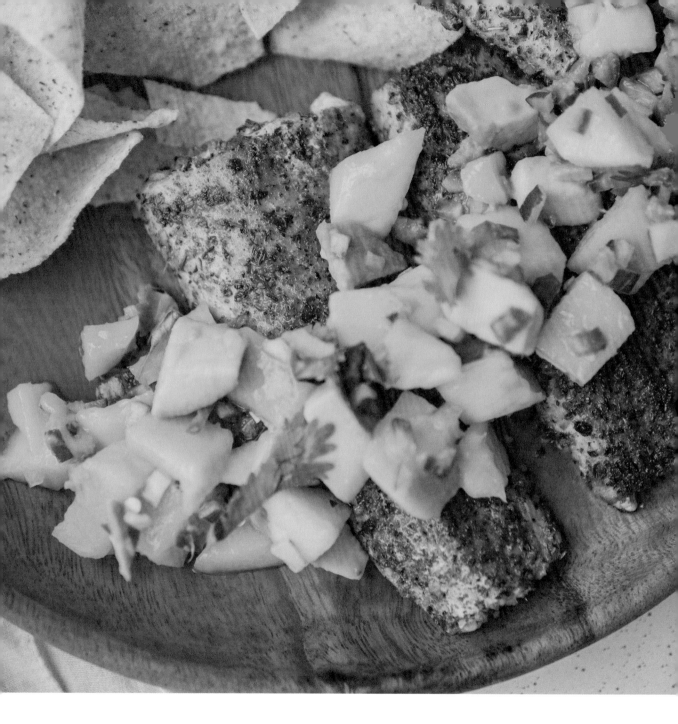

CRISPY COD WITH MALT VINEGAR-ROASTED POTATOES & MALT-MINT PEA CHIMI

SERVES: 4
PREP TIME: 20 MINUTES
COOK TIME: 45 MINUTES

2 pounds Yukon Gold potatoes, halved

1½ cups water

½ cup malt vinegar, divided

½ cup olive oil, divided

1 teaspoon black pepper

1 cup all-purpose flour

½ cup white cornmeal

2 teaspoons Old Bay

1 teaspoon garlic powder

2 eggs

4–6 skinless cod fillets

Kosher salt and freshly ground pepper to taste

Malt-Mint Pea Chimi for serving (see recipe on page 118)

Sweet Heat Tartar Sauce (see recipe on page 118)

THIS IS not a seasonal dish by any means, but growing up, we'd go for "fish and chips" in the summertime, so I can't help but relate it back to the days of salty beach skin and sand. I've tied together the New England flavors I grew up with, like malt vinegar, with the traditional British pairings of peas and mint. Bright and crisp flavors while being a hearty and filling meal to end the day.

Preheat the oven to 425°F/220°C.

Place the potatoes cut-side down on a large rimmed baking sheet. Pour the water over the potatoes and add ¼ cup of malt vinegar. Cover the baking sheet tightly with aluminum foil. Roast for 20–25 minutes or until fork tender. Carefully, lift one edge of the aluminum foil and drain the water from the tray. Remove the aluminum foil completely.

Drizzle the potatoes with 2 tablespoons of olive oil, sprinkle with black pepper, and toss to coat. Return the potatoes, uncovered, to the oven to roast an additional 20–25 minutes until golden.

While the potatoes roast, heat a heavy-bottomed pot or cast-iron skillet over medium heat. Pour the remaining olive oil into the skillet to heat. This should only be about a ¼ inch of oil in the skillet for a shallow fry.

In a shallow dish, combine flour, cornmeal, Old Bay, and garlic powder. In a separate dish, whisk the eggs.

Pat the cod fillets dry with a paper towel. Lightly season the flesh of the fish with salt and pepper. Dredge the fish in the egg and then the flour mixture to fully coat, shaking off any excess.

Cook the fish in the hot oil for 3–4 minutes on each side or until lightly browned and the internal temperature reaches 135–140°F/57–60°C. Place on a paper towel–lined plate and set aside until ready to serve.

Serve the fried fish with potatoes, drizzled in the remaining malt vinegar along with the Malt-Mint Pea Chimi and Sweet Heat Tartar Sauce.

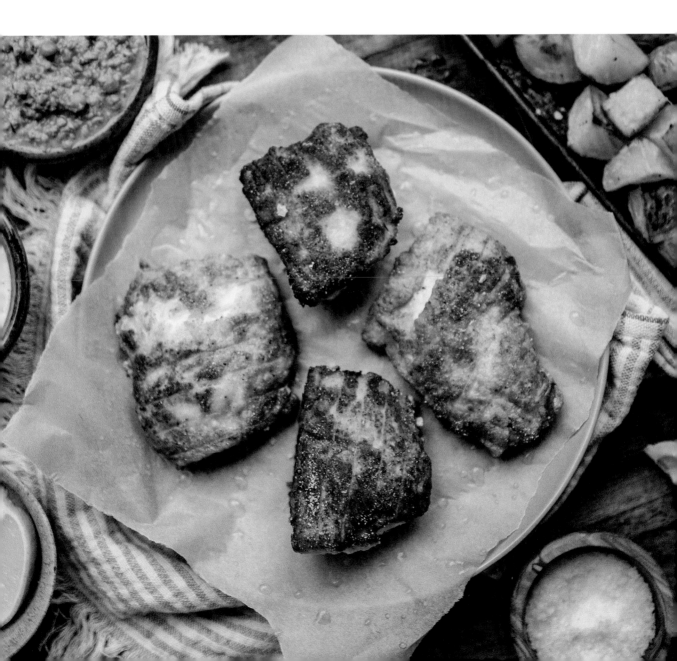

MALT-MINT PEA CHIMI

YIELDS: ABOUT 2 CUPS
PREP TIME: 5 MINUTES
COOK TIME: 0 MINUTES

¼ cup malt vinegar

2 tablespoons honey

1 teaspoon garlic, minced

¼ cup fresh mint leaves

3 tablespoons olive oil

2 cups peas, divided (frozen and thawed are best, canned peas are not as fresh)

Salt and pepper to taste

In a food processor, add malt vinegar, honey, garlic, mint, and olive oil. Blitz for 30 seconds until smooth. Add half the peas and blitz for 10–15 seconds until slightly broken down. Add the mix to a medium bowl, combine the remaining peas, and stir to combine. Taste and adjust salt and pepper as needed. Cover and refrigerate until ready to serve.

SWEET HEAT TARTAR SAUCE

YIELDS: ABOUT 1¼ CUPS
PREP TIME: 5 MINUTES
COOK TIME: 0 MINUTES

1 cup mayonnaise

½ cup bread-and-butter pickles, minced

2 tablespoons yellow onion, minced

1 tablespoon capers, drained and minced

1 tablespoon fresh parsley, minced

1 tablespoon lemon juice

½ teaspoon pepper

¼ teaspoon kosher salt

¼ teaspoon cayenne pepper

Mix all ingredients in a small bowl, cover, and refrigerate until ready to serve.

ROASTED COD, BURSTING SUMMER TOMATOES, SWEET CORN & CRISPY PROSCIUTTO

SERVES: 4
PREP TIME: 10 MINUTES
COOK TIME: 35 MINUTES

2 ears sweet corn, husked

¼ cup olive oil, divided

Pinch salt

3 tablespoons Piri Piri Sauce (see page 60 for recipe)

1 tablespoon sherry vinegar

1 tablespoon tomato paste

1 teaspoon honey

½ teaspoon ground cumin

2 garlic cloves, grated

1½ pounds skin-on cod

Salt and pepper to taste

2 pints mini heirloom tomatoes

8 ounces prosciutto

Parsley leaves for garnish

Lemon wedge for serving

COD WAS not a fish I grew up enjoying, and boy, was I missing out. We absolutely love cod for its subtle buttery flavor and flaky flesh. This cod dish is the perfect balance of sweet from the fresh summer vegetables, spicy from the sauce, and salty from the added prosciutto. Set this pan down in the middle of the table and let your guests eat with their eyes first!

Preheat the oven to 400°F/200°C.

On a large baking sheet, lay the corn, drizzle with 1 tablespoon of olive oil and a pinch of salt. Roast for 15 minutes.

In a medium bowl, mix the Piri Piri sauce, 2 tablespoons of olive oil, vinegar, tomato paste, honey, cumin, and garlic to make the red pepper sauce.

Place the cod on a baking sheet. Season with salt and pepper. Lightly cover the cod with the red pepper sauce, reserving a few tablespoons for serving. Toss the mini heirloom tomatoes with the remaining tablespoon of olive oil and salt. Lay the tomatoes around the cod. Place pieces of prosciutto on top of the tomatoes. Roast for 15–20 minutes or until the internal temperature of the cod reaches 140°F/60°C.

When ready to serve, cut the corn off the cobs and toss with the tomatoes. Top with the reserved red pepper sauce, parsley, and a squeeze of lemon.

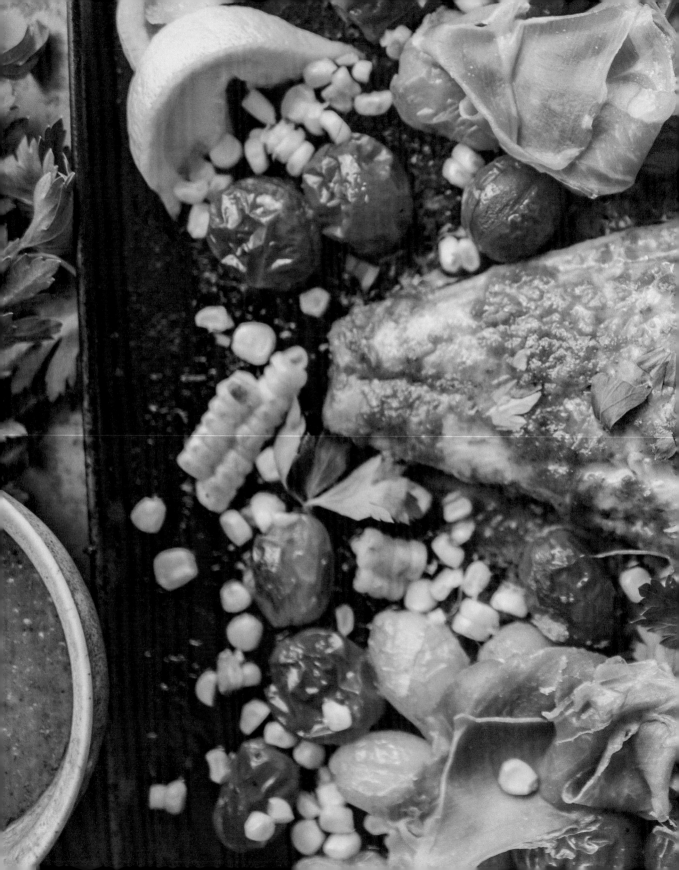

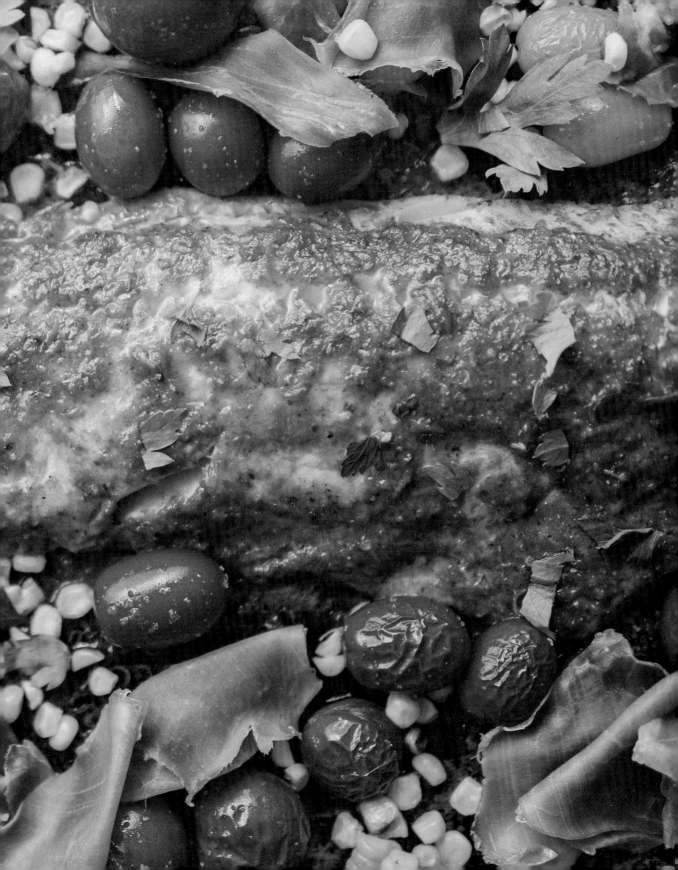

SIMPLE SHRIMP BOIL FOIL PACKETS

SERVES: 4

PREP TIME: 10 MINUTES

COOK TIME: 30 MINUTES

1 pound baby potatoes, halved

2 ears sweet corn, husked, sliced into rounds

2 pounds easy-peel shrimp (peeled works great too!)

1 sweet onion, thickly sliced

1 pound andouille sausage, sliced into ½-inch pieces

2 tablespoons olive oil

2 teaspoons Old Bay seasoning

12 ounces light Mexican beer

6 tablespoons salted butter

Fresh parsley chopped for serving

FOIL PACKET dinners make for the easiest cleanup, and I'm all about it. These are classic flavors reminiscent of summer days by the New England coast. Comforting potatoes and sweet summer corn with tangy Mexican beer and Old Bay–spiced shrimp all rolled into a personal packet will leave the family, or your dinner guests, raving about this meal. Not to mention this is a super-simple, ten-ingredient recipe. Winner, winner, Old Bay shrimp for dinner!

Add the potatoes to a large pot of salted water, bring to a rolling boil, and cook for 6–10 minutes until tender. Drain and set aside.

Preheat the oven to 400°F/200°C.

On a large baking sheet, toss the potatoes, corn, shrimp, onion, and sausage with olive oil and sprinkle with Old Bay until everything is evenly coated.

Tear four sheets of aluminum foil and four sheets of parchment paper. Lay a sheet of parchment paper on each sheet of aluminum foil. Crimp the sides to create a small bowl. Evenly distribute the potatoes, corn, onion, and shrimp to each parchment-lined foil sheet. Seal the sides together, and just before fully closing the packet, pour 3 ounces of Mexican beer into each packet.

Tightly close the packets, place on a large baking sheet, and bake in the oven for 15–18 minutes.

While the foil packets are cooking, heat a small saucepan over medium heat. Add the 6 tablespoons of salted butter to the pan and cook until frothy, fragrant, and brown. Remove from the heat and set aside until ready to serve.

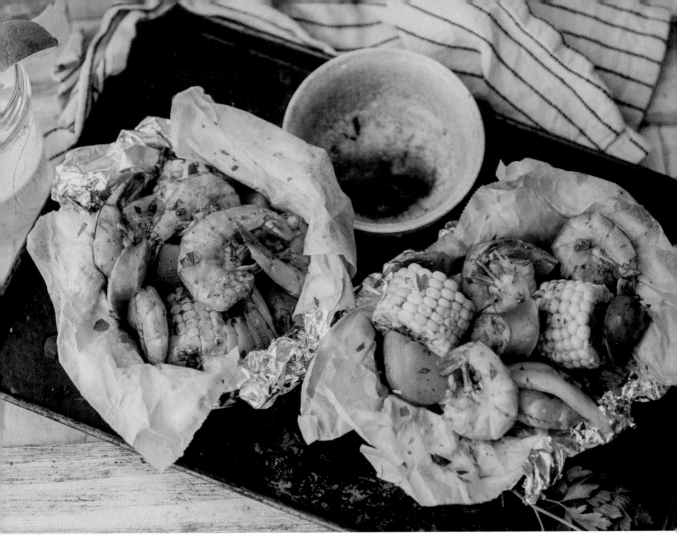

Remove the foil packets from the oven, carefully opening each to release the steam. Drizzle each packet with browned butter and sprinkle with fresh chopped parsley. Serve immediately with cold Mexican beer.

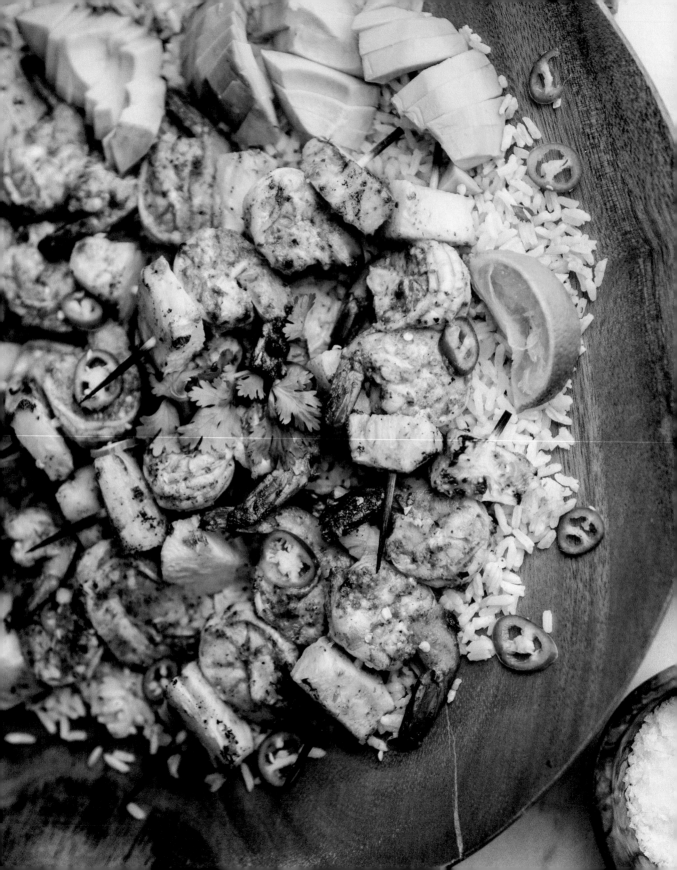

POBLANO SHRIMP & PINEAPPLE SKEWERS

SERVES: 4

PREP TIME: 45 MINUTES

COOK TIME: 10 MINUTES

½ cup extra-virgin olive oil

½ cup sour orange juice

⅓ cup fresh lime juice

½ cup cilantro leaves and stems

2 tablespoons fresh mint leaves

4 garlic cloves

1 teaspoon oregano

2 teaspoons ground cumin

½ teaspoon salt

½ teaspoon pepper

¼ teaspoon red pepper flakes

2 poblano peppers, roasted and divided

2 cups fresh pineapple, cubed

2 pounds raw shrimp, peeled and deveined

Steamed white rice or Jalapeño-Lime-Coconut White Rice (see page 140 for recipe)

2 ripe avocados, sliced for serving

Serrano peppers, sliced for serving

Cilantro for serving

I LOVE how simple this shrimp dish is to put together, and yet it's bright and flavorful. The shrimp absorbs the strong citrus flavor like a champ, and the cilantro and mint bring a brightness to balance out the heat from the poblanos. Put the kids to work on this one, and recruit their little hands to build their own skewers. Time to get your hands into the mess and make this dish for your next meal!

Place the first twelve ingredients into a blender or food processor, process for about 1 minute or until smooth.

Reserve ½ cup of marinade for serving. Transfer the remaining marinade to a large bowl and add the shrimp, toss to coat. Cover and refrigerate for 30 minutes.

Preheat the grill to 450–500°F/230–260°C. Build the skewers, alternating with pineapple and shrimp. Grill until the shrimp is bright pink and lightly charred, about 2–3 minutes per side.

Serve hot over a bed of rice drizzled with the reserved marinade along with avocado, serrano peppers, and cilantro.

SEAFOOD

KICKIN' CASHEW SHRIMP BOWLS

SERVES: 4
PREP TIME: 10 MINUTES
COOK TIME: 25 MINUTES

1 tablespoon olive oil

1 cup cashews, dry roasted

2 tablespoons Sweet Chili Sauce (see page 77 for recipe), divided

1 teaspoon orange zest

Pinch flaky salt

1 teaspoon sesame seeds, plus more for serving

2 pounds raw peeled shrimp

¼ cup white cornmeal

¼ teaspoon salt

¼ teaspoon pepper

2–4 tablespoons olive oil

¼ cup soy sauce

3 tablespoons rice vinegar

3 tablespoons ketchup

1 teaspoon sesame oil

1 teaspoon garlic, grated

½ teaspoon fresh ginger, grated

Steamed white rice

¼ cup scallions, diced for garnish

THIS IS soon to become your new favorite meal made in under 40 minutes. It comes together in a flash, and shrimp for dinner always feels a little fancy. Put the take-away menus down and do yourself a favor by whipping up this fancy and flavorful dish with kickin' cashews and saucy shrimp.

Heat the olive oil in a large cast-iron skillet over medium heat. When the oil shimmers, add the cashews and 1 tablespoon of Sweet Chili Sauce. Cook until lightly toasted, about 3–4 minutes. Move the cashews to a parchment-lined plate, sprinkle with orange zest, salt, and sesame seeds, and set aside.

Lay the shrimp on a paper towel–lined baking sheet to remove excess surface moisture. In a large bowl, whisk the white cornmeal, salt, and pepper. Toss the shrimp with the seasoned cornmeal to coat. Shake off any excess flour before cooking.

Heat the same skillet with 2 tablespoons of olive oil over medium heat. Working in batches, cook the shrimp for 2–3 minutes on each side. Move the cooked shrimp to a plate or baking tray while you finish cooking the remaining shrimp.

Meanwhile, whisk the soy sauce, rice vinegar, ketchup, sesame oil, garlic, ginger, and remaining tablespoon of Sweet Chili Sauce in a small bowl. Return all the cooked shrimp to the skillet, reduce the heat to low, and pour the sauce over the shrimp. Simmer for 3–5 minutes until the sauce has slightly thickened.

Serve the shrimp over a bed of steamed rice, topped with kickin' cashews, scallions, and sesame seeds.

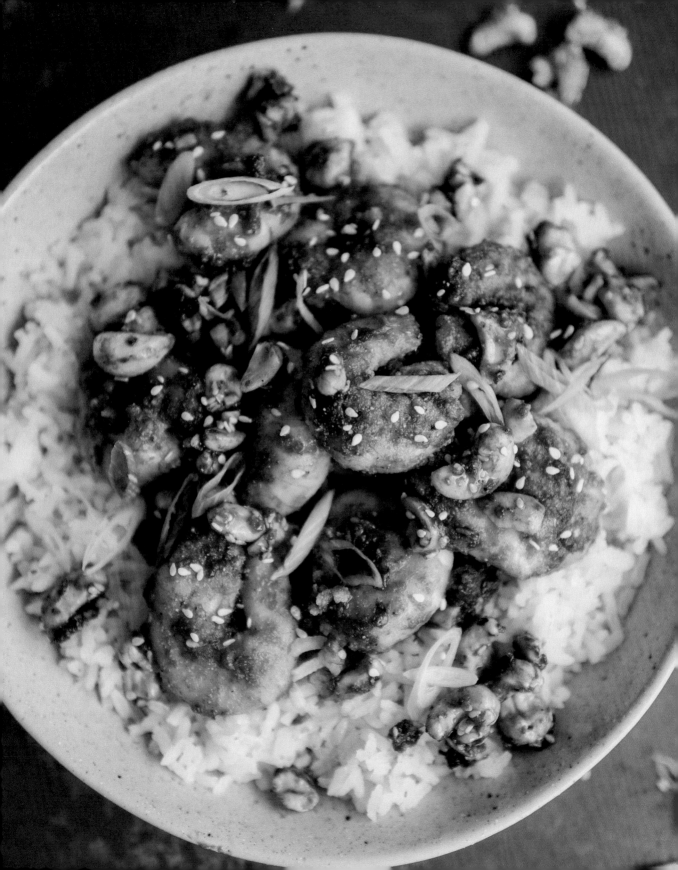

HORSERADISH SALMON WITH ROASTED ASPARAGUS

SERVES: 4
PREP TIME: 5 MINUTES
COOK TIME: 12 MINUTES

4 wild-caught salmon fillets

Pinch of kosher salt

¼ cup mayonnaise

1 tablespoon horseradish

1 tablespoon fresh parsley, minced

1 cup panko

2 large bunches of asparagus, woody ends removed

1 tablespoon olive oil

Salt and pepper to taste

Lemon wedge for serving

WE ALL have those busy nights where dinner seems like an impossible task. We want something quick but don't want to sacrifice quality and flavor. Do you have 20 minutes to spare? If the answer is "YES," then this recipe is for you. The longest part of this recipe is likely waiting on the oven to preheat!

Preheat the oven to 350°F/177°C.

Lay the salmon fillets on an aluminum foil-lined baking sheet. Season each fillet with a pinch or two of salt. In a small bowl, whisk mayonnaise, horseradish, and minced parsley. Evenly distribute the horseradish mixture to the tops of each salmon fillet. Sprinkle each fillet with ¼ cup of panko, lightly pressing the panko into the horseradish mixture. Lay the crusted salmon on the aluminum foil-lined baking sheet with room in between each fillet.

Between the fillets of salmon, lay the asparagus. Drizzle the asparagus with olive oil and lightly season with salt and pepper.

Roast in the oven for 10–12 minutes or until the internal temperature of the salmon reaches 120°F/48°C.

Serve each fillet with a side of asparagus and a lemon wedge.

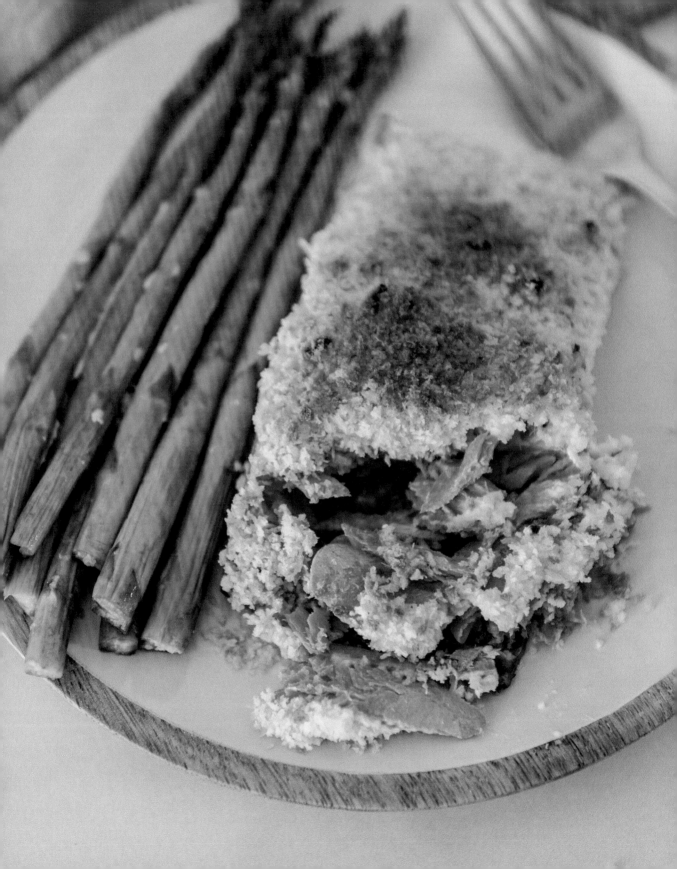

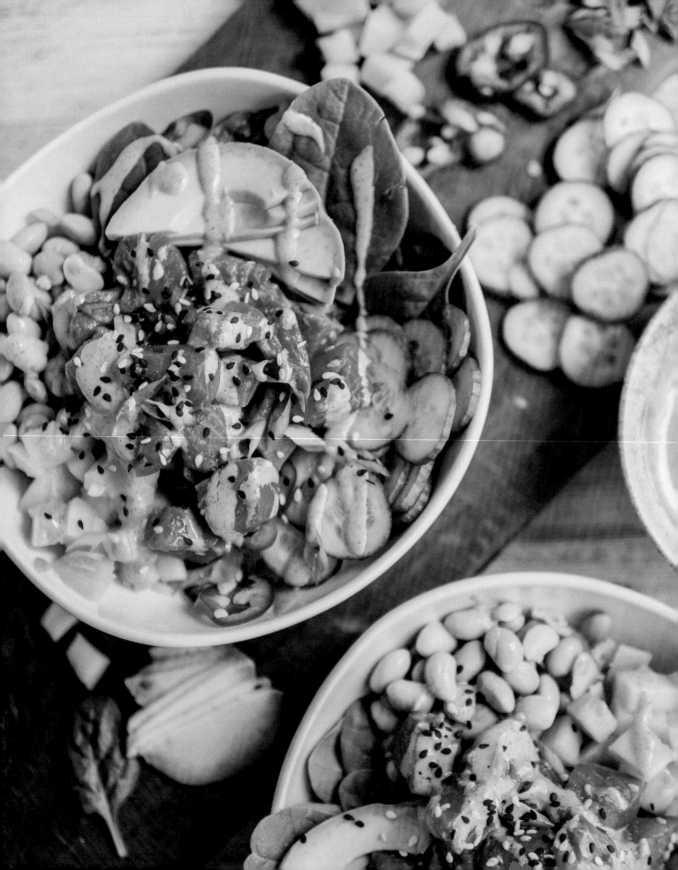

ZESTY ORANGE SALMON POKÉ BOWLS

SERVES: 4
PREP TIME: 40 MINUTES
COOK TIME: 0 MINUTES

¼ cup tamari (or soy sauce)

¼ cup orange juice plus 1 teaspoon orange zest

2 tablespoons lime juice

1 tablespoon sambal oelek (can be found in the international aisle at most grocery stores)

2 teaspoons toasted sesame oil

2 tablespoons white sesame seeds, toasted and divided

1 teaspoon maple syrup

1 pound sushi-grade salmon, cubed

¼ cup mayonnaise

1–2 tablespoons sriracha

1 cup steamed white rice

1 cup spinach

1 cup shelled edamame

2 cups persian cucumbers, sliced thin

2 ripe mangos, diced

1 ripe avocado, sliced

1 jalapeño, sliced

1 tablespoon black sesame seeds, toasted

2 green onions, sliced

POKÉ BOWLS used to be a meal we'd get while traveling along the coast. Our longing for these bowls urged me to hunt down the freshest fish I could find and re-create them at home. I don't know why I waited so long! These bowls are fresh, flavorful, and just spicy enough to leave a tingle on your tongue. The heat is tamed by fresh bursts of mango and avocado and pops of edamame.

In a large bowl, whisk tamari, orange juice, orange zest, lime juice, sambal oelek, sesame oil, 1 tablespoon of sesame seeds, and maple syrup. To the bowl add the cubed salmon. Toss to fully coat, cover and refrigerate for at least 30 minutes.

In a small bowl, whisk the mayonnaise and sriracha. Set aside until ready to assemble.

To assemble the poké bowl, start with a base of white rice and spinach. Add edamame, cucumbers, mangos, avocado slices, and jalapeños. Top each bowl with a heaping scoop of salmon. Drizzle with the sriracha mayo and sprinkle with white and black sesame seeds and green onions.

SEAFOOD

SMOKED SALMON BURGERS WITH CRISP SLAW

SERVES: 4

PREP TIME: 15 MINUTES

COOK TIME: 15 MINUTES

2 cups green cabbage, shredded

1 cup fresh parsley, chopped

½ cup celery, thinly sliced

3 tablespoons capers, drained and minced

3 tablespoons red wine vinegar

3 tablespoons olive oil

Salt and pepper to taste

16 ounces smoked salmon (see page 135 for recipe)

2 eggs

½ cup panko

2 tablespoons fresh parsley

2 tablespoons fresh dill

1 teaspoon lemon juice

1 teaspoon salt

½ teaspoon garlic powder

1–2 tablespoons olive oil

Flaky salt

3 tablespoons Sweet Heat Tartar Sauce (see page 118 for recipe)

HOT-SMOKED SALMON can be found in most grocery stores. *Hot-smoked* means the salmon is cooked through and flaky versus *cold-smoked*, which is silky and resembles lox from a fancy brunch buffet. If you don't have a smoker of your own, feel free to swap in high-quality, store-bought hot-smoked salmon, and this recipe will come together in a breeze.

In a large bowl, mix the cabbage, parsley, celery, capers, red wine vinegar, and olive oil. Taste and season with salt and pepper accordingly. Cover and refrigerate until ready to serve.

In a large bowl, mix the salmon, eggs, panko, parsley, dill, lemon juice, salt, and garlic powder. Divide the salmon mixture into 4–6 patties and flatten slightly between your palms. Set a cast-iron skillet on the stove over medium heat and add 1–2 tablespoons of olive oil. When the oil shimmers, add the salmon patties, working in batches if needed so you do not crowd the pan. Fry on each side 2–3 minutes or until golden. Move the cooked patties to a paper towel-lined plate and sprinkle with flaky salt.

Serve each patty on top of the crispy cabbage slaw, topped with a dollop of tartar sauce.

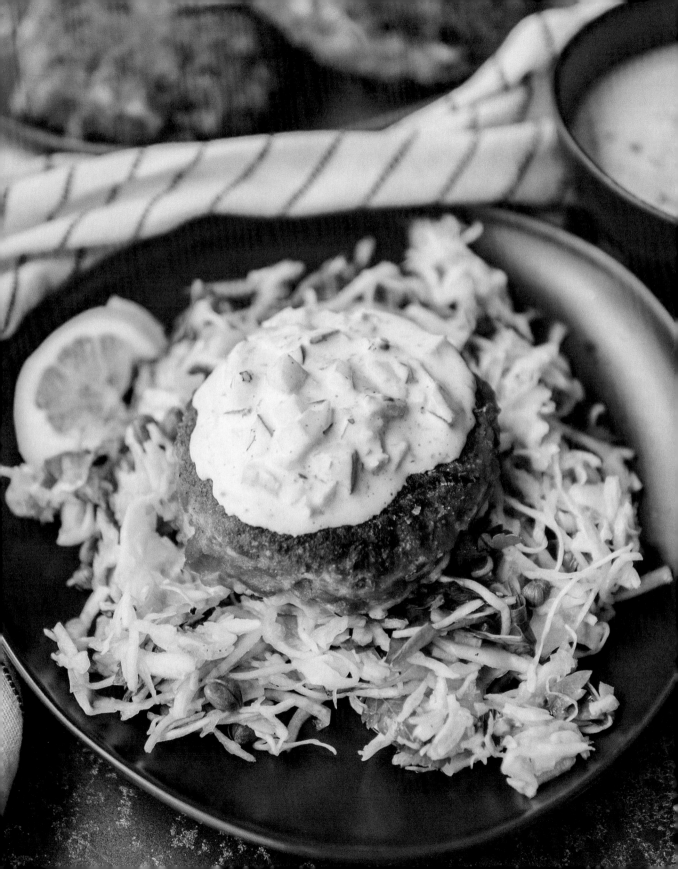

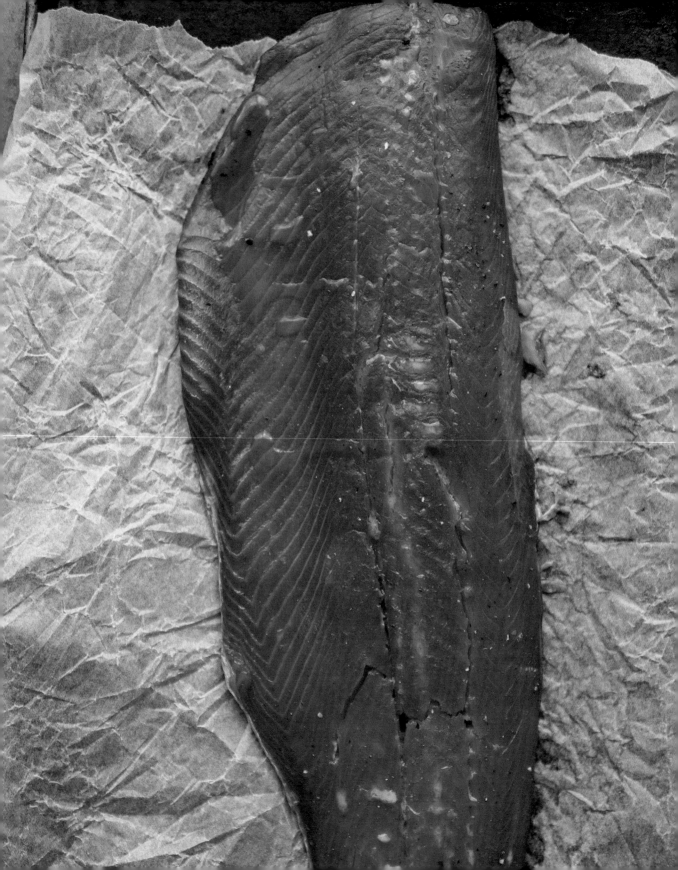

HOT-SMOKED SALMON

SERVES: 4

PREP TIME: 35 MINUTES (PLUS 2 HOURS MARINATING)

COOK TIME: 90 MINUTES

3 tablespoons kosher salt

Zest of 2 lemons

1 teaspoon ground black pepper

2 tablespoons maple syrup

2 tablespoons vodka

2½ pounds wild-caught Alaskan salmon fillet with skin

HOT-SMOKED SALMON is much smokier and has a baked flakiness to the fish, whereas cold smoked salmon is less smoky, and silky. Cold-smoked salmon texture is similar to that of lox. I absolutely love the texture of hot-smoked salmon, and the smoky flavor is exactly what I'm looking for in a smoked salmon.

Line a 9x13 glass baking dish with a large piece of cling wrap (this will be used to wrap the salmon, so make sure it's big enough!). In a small bowl, mix the salt, lemon zest, and pepper with your hands until the lemon is fragrant. Add the maple syrup and vodka, and mix until it resembles a paste.

Pat the salmon fillet dry with paper towels, then press the paste into the flesh of the salmon. Place the salmon flesh-side down on the cling wrap. Wrap it tightly and rest in the glass baking dish in the refrigerator for 2 hours. Remove the salmon from the fridge, discard the cling wrap, and rinse the cure from the salmon. Pat the salmon dry and rest on a wire rack above a baking sheet on the counter for 30 minutes.

While the salmon is air drying, preheat the smoker. Set the Traeger Grill to "Smoke" or 180°F/82°C. Smoke the salmon for 45 minutes. Increase the temperature to 225°F/107°C and cook for an additional 30–40 minutes or until the internal temperature reaches 120°F/48°C. Allow the salmon to cool for 10–15 minutes before lightly shredding with a fork.

AHI TUNA TACOS

SERVES: 4
PREP TIME: 40 MINUTES
COOK TIME: 10 MINUTES

1 cup radish, thinly sliced

¼ cup red onion, thinly sliced

¼ cup lime juice

2 teaspoons kosher salt

2 pounds ahi tuna steaks

¼ cup tamari (or soy sauce), divided

¼ cup mayonnaise

¼ cup sriracha

1 cup green cabbage, shredded

2 tablespoons hoisin sauce

1 tablespoon hot water

1 tablespoon olive oil

1 tablespoon white toasted sesame seeds

1 tablespoon black toasted sesame seeds

1 tablespoon furikake seasoning, optional

Serrano pepper, thinly sliced

12 street taco–size flour tortillas, fire-roasted**

IF YOU ask the Well-Fed Fraser what he's feeling for dinner, 99 percent of the time he'll pause and then say, "Tacos." The most amazing thing about that answer is you can empty the fridge into a flour or corn tortilla and call it a taco. These Ahi Tuna Tacos were a showstopper, and while they may look fancy, these are some of the simplest tacos to make. Believe it or not, most of the legwork is in the assembly! Once you've got all the components laid out on fire-roasted tortillas, these tacos will be gone before you know it!

In a medium bowl or jar, combine the radish, red onion, lime juice, and kosher salt. Mix to fully incorporate, cover, and refrigerate for at least 30 minutes.

In a separate medium bowl, place the ahi tuna steak and 3 tablespoons of tamari. Flip the steaks around in the bowl to coat in the tamari. Cover and refrigerate for at least 30 minutes.

While you're waiting for the radish and tuna to marinate, prepare your other ingredients. In a medium bowl, whisk together mayonnaise and sriracha. Add the shredded green cabbage and toss to dress. Cover and refrigerate until ready to serve.

In a small dish, whisk together the remaining tablespoon of tamari with the hoisin and hot water. Set aside until ready to serve.

Remove the tuna from the fridge. Heat olive oil in a large skillet over medium heat. In a shallow dish, combine the white and black toasted sesame seeds. Press the tuna steaks into the seeds to create a crust on the tuna and then place them into the hot pan. Sear on each

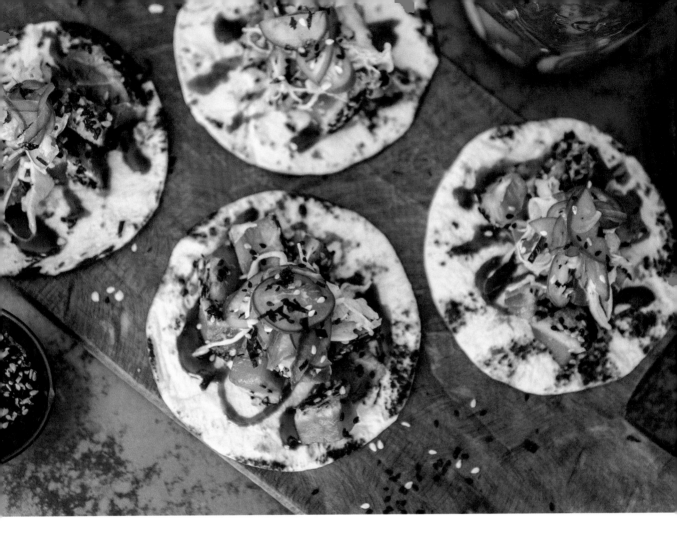

side for 2–3 minutes. Remove from the heat and place on a clean plate. Work in batches if needed. Slice and cube the tuna for serving.

To assemble the tacos, drizzle 1–2 teaspoons of the hoisin sauce on each fire-roasted tortilla. Top with cubed tuna, sriracha cabbage, furikake, serrano peppers, and lime-pickled radish and onions.

** This can easily be done on a gas stove over the open flame for 20–30 seconds per side. Watch carefully, as they will burn quickly. Flip constantly until desired doneness. If you have an electric stove, you can toast your tortillas in a skillet over medium heat, flipping constantly until desired doneness.

SEAFOOD

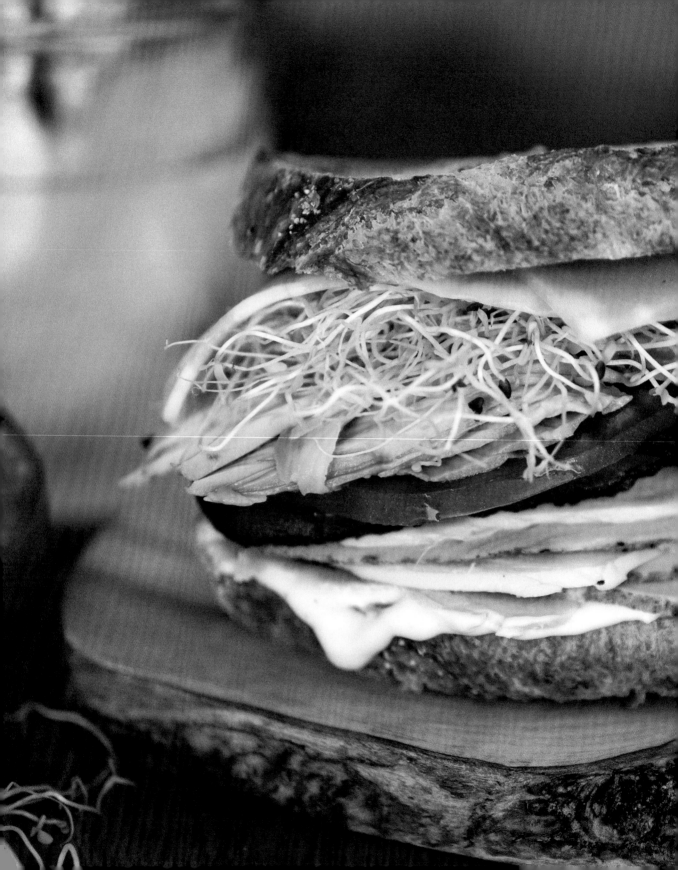

SIDES, SALADS & SANDWICHES

JALAPEÑO-LIME-COCONUT WHITE RICE

SERVES: 8–10
PREP TIME: 5 MINUTES
COOK TIME: 40 MINUTES

1 cup full-fat coconut milk

1 jalapeño, roughly chopped and seeded for less spice

½ cup cilantro stems

2 tablespoons salted butter

2 cups basmati/jasmine rice

2½ cups water

1 teaspoon fresh cracked pepper

Pinch salt

¼ cup cilantro leaves, chopped for garnish

¼ cup lime juice

THIS IS a kickin' version of my classic white rice recipe. If you want the original, simply take out the cilantro, jalapeños, and lime from the recipe below and you'll be left with a simple Coconut White Rice that pairs well with *any* recipe. For those of you who like a little kick with your meal, this is the rice recipe for you!

In a blender or food processor, blitz the coconut milk, jalapeño, and cilantro stems for 30–60 seconds. Set aside.

In a medium saucepan, melt 2 tablespoons of salted butter over high heat. Just as the butter melts, add the uncooked rice. Stir to coat the rice in the butter, and toast for 1 minute. Add the water and jalapeño coconut milk, black pepper, and salt. Bring the rice to a rolling boil, then reduce the heat to low, cover, and cook for 20 minutes.

When the timer rings, turn the heat off, but leave the pot covered on the stove for an additional 20 minutes to rest.

Before serving, add the chopped cilantro leaves and lime juice. Toss to incorporate.

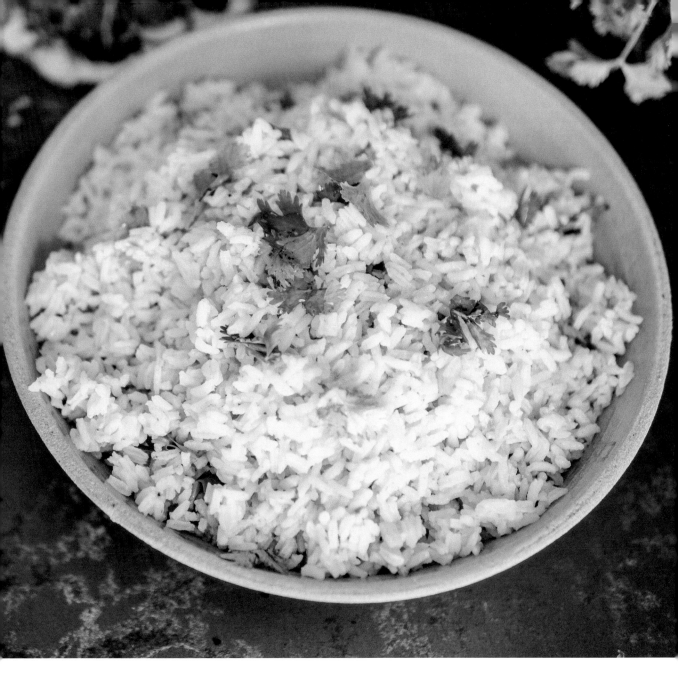

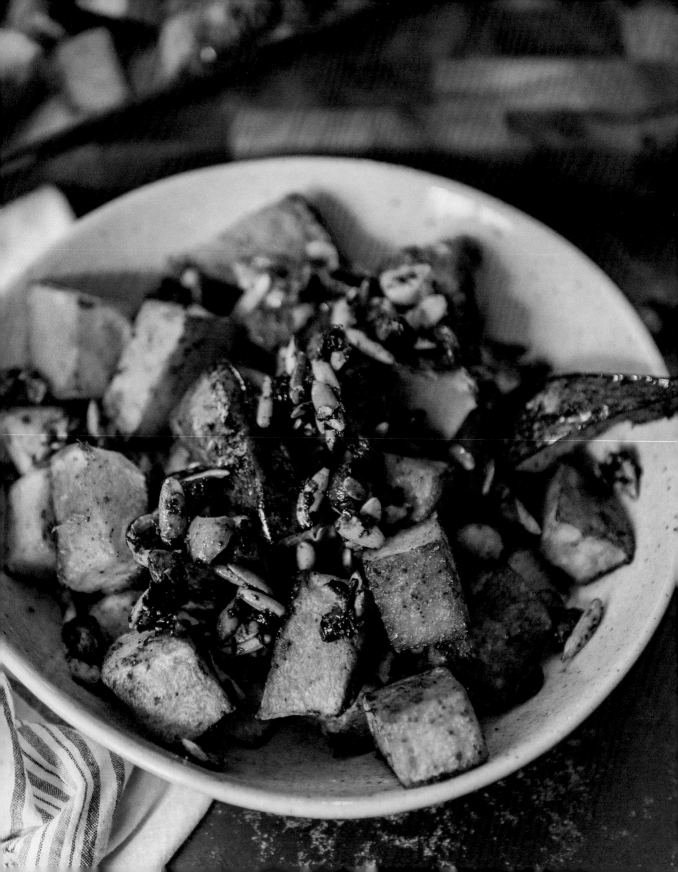

ROASTED BUTTERNUT & ACORN SQUASH WITH MIXED-NUT CRUMBLE

SERVES: 4–6
PREP TIME: 15 MINUTES
COOK TIME: 75 MINUTES

¼ cup salted butter

⅔ cup pepitas

½ cup raw hazelnuts, roughly chopped

¼ cup pistachios

¼ cup maple syrup, divided

1 teaspoon cinnamon

Pinch flaky salt

¼ cup olive oil

1 tablespoon chili powder

2 teaspoons cumin

4 cups butternut squash, peeled and cut into 2-inch pieces

2 cups acorn squash, quartered lengthwise

OUR TWO favorite fall vegetables are butternut and acorn squash. By mid-October, I've likely pulled all the fall sweaters into my closet and made some form of roasted squash at least once a week. Enjoy this simple roasted squash with warm spiced and crunchy nut crumble as a side to any weeknight dinner, or toss with leafy greens to make a roasted squash side salad. Perfect for the holiday season!

To make the mixed-nut crumble, preheat the oven to 350°F/177°C. Line a baking sheet with parchment paper and set aside.

In a small sauté pan over medium heat, melt ¼ cup of butter. Cook, stirring constantly, for about 2 minutes until the butter is foamy and browned. Remove from the heat and pour the butter into a large bowl with the pepitas, hazelnuts, pistachios, 2 tablespoons of maple syrup, and cinnamon. Toss to combine. Lay the mixture evenly out on the baking sheet and sprinkle with a pinch or two of flaky salt. Roast in the preheated oven for 20–25 minutes, tossing every 10 minutes to ensure an even cook. Remove from the oven and set aside to cool.

Increase the oven temperature to 400°F/200°C.

In a small bowl, mix the olive oil, remaining 2 tablespoons of maple syrup, chili powder, and cumin. Lay the butternut squash and acorn squash onto two parchment-lined baking sheets. Drizzle with the oil-and-spice mixture, tossing with your hands to fully coat. Roast the squash for 25 minutes. Flip the squash and roast for an additional 20 minutes or until golden brown.

Remove the squash from the oven to cool slightly. Top the roasted squash with the mixed-nut crumble before serving.

MUSTARD-ROASTED POTATOES & ASPARAGUS

SERVES: 4
PREP TIME: 10 MINUTES
COOK TIME: 35–40 MINUTES

1 pound baby Yukon Gold
or fingerling potatoes,
quartered

1 tablespoon olive oil

Salt and pepper

1 bunch asparagus, woody
ends trimmed, cut into
2-inch pieces

2 tablespoons whole-grain
mustard

1 tablespoon white balsamic
vinegar

½ teaspoon red pepper
flakes

2 teaspoons (or to taste)
flaky salt

IT'S SO easy to fall into a vegetable side dish rut. Steamed broccoli and simple roasted asparagus have a special place in my heart and serve a purpose for many meals, *but* I'm trying to keep mealtime exciting. The best part about a side dish like this is not only is it exciting for your taste buds but it's simple to make!

Preheat the Traeger Grill (or oven) to 400°F/200°C. Toss the potatoes with olive oil and season with salt and pepper. Place the seasoned potatoes on a large baking sheet and roast for 20 minutes. Flip the potatoes and add the asparagus to the tray. Roast an additional 10–15 minutes until the potatoes are browned and the asparagus is cooked but still crunchy.

In a small bowl, mix the whole-grain mustard, balsamic vinegar, and red pepper flakes. Pour the mustard dressing over the potatoes and asparagus. Toss to combine. Taste and add flaky finishing salt to taste. Serve immediately. See page 167 to add these Mustard-Roasted Potatoes & Asparagus to an herby salad!

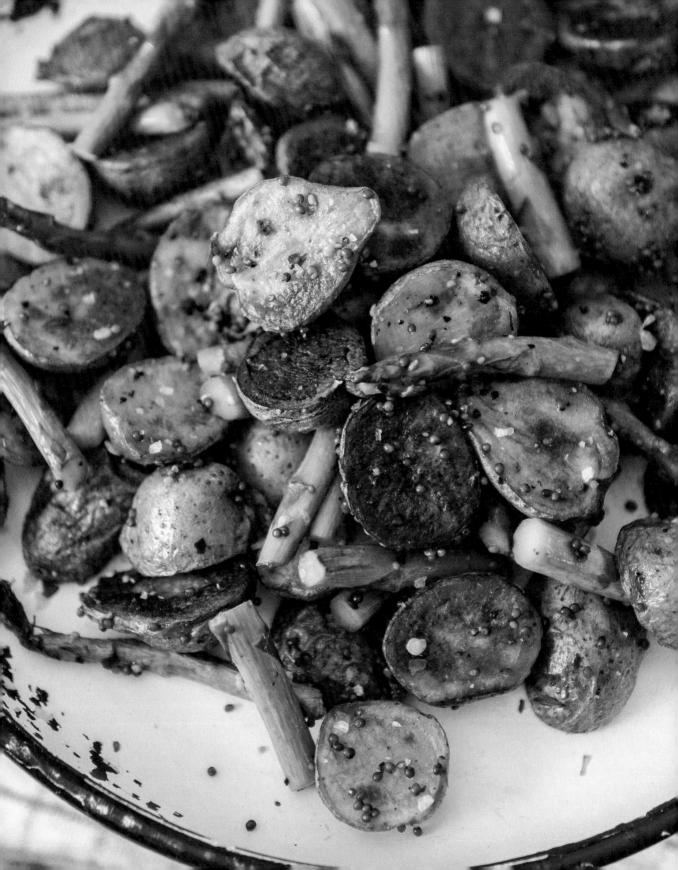

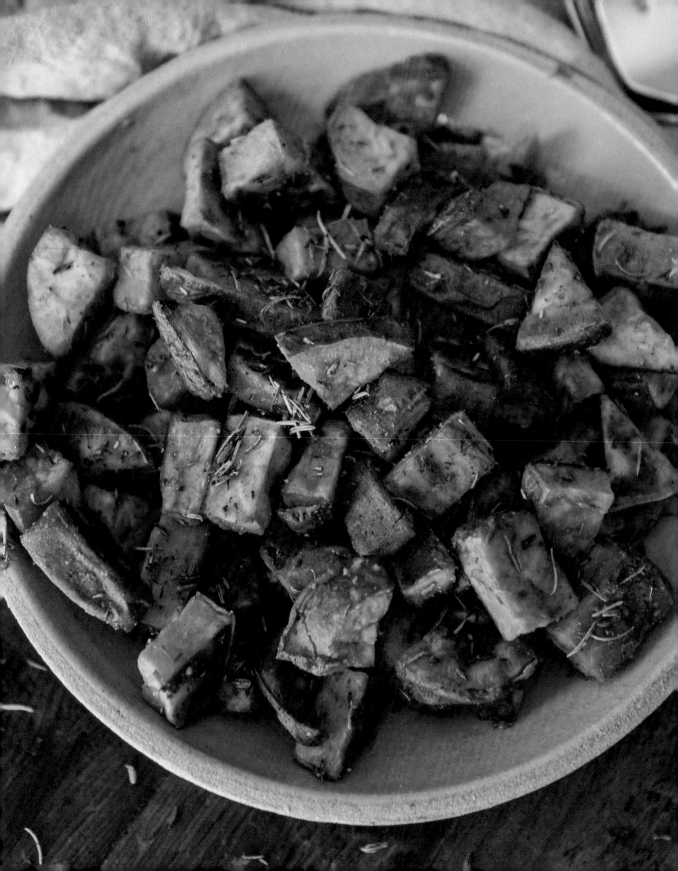

FENNEL-ROASTED SWEET POTATOES

SERVES: 4
PREP TIME: 10 MINUTES
COOK TIME: 40 MINUTES

2 teaspoons salt

2 teaspoons fennel seeds

2 teaspoons garlic

2 teaspoons rosemary

1 teaspoon thyme

½ teaspoon sage

4 large sweet potatoes, cubed

2 tablespoons olive oil

THIS SPICE mix is most commonly used on ribs in our house. After making a double batch of the rub one weekend for ribs, I had a container lingering on my counter during a day of meal prepping. In an effort to make simple roasted sweet potatoes a little more exciting, I sprinkled a heavy hand of this seasoning on them before roasting. The bold spice flavors pair well with the subtly sweet root vegetable.

Preheat the oven to 425°F/220°C. In a small bowl, mix the spices. Lay the sweet potatoes out on two baking sheets to allow enough space between them for crisping. Drizzle each sheet with olive oil and evenly distribute the spice mix. Toss with your hands and space the potatoes out.

Roast for 20 minutes. Remove from the oven, toss, and roast for an additional 15–20 minutes until lightly browned and crisp.

SIDES, SALADS & SANDWICHES

SMOKED TOMATOES

YIELDS: ABOUT 1 CUP
PREP TIME: 5 MINUTES
COOK TIME: 2 HOURS

2 pints cherry tomatoes,
halved

4 tablespoons olive oil

2 teaspoons flaky salt

NO SMOKER on your back porch? No fear! You can make this recipe in the oven using the same temperature and time. Whenever I've got to slow cook anything for 2-plus hours, you can bet it's either a weekend project or something I'll make the night before, while that evening's dinner is in motion, to reheat the next day. These smoked (or slow-roasted) tomatoes store well in an airtight container and are reheated either on the stove top or a quick zap in the microwave.

Preheat the Traeger Grill to 300°F/150°C. Spread the tomatoes into one layer on a baking sheet and drizzle with the olive oil. Toss and sprinkle with flaky salt. Place into the smoker to roast for 2 hours. Serve on toast (see page 9 for the Smoked Tomatoes, Whipped Ricotta & Fried Eggs recipe), in a sandwich (see page 171 for Smoky BLT recipe), add to pasta salad, or mix into a homemade pasta sauce for an elevated flavor.

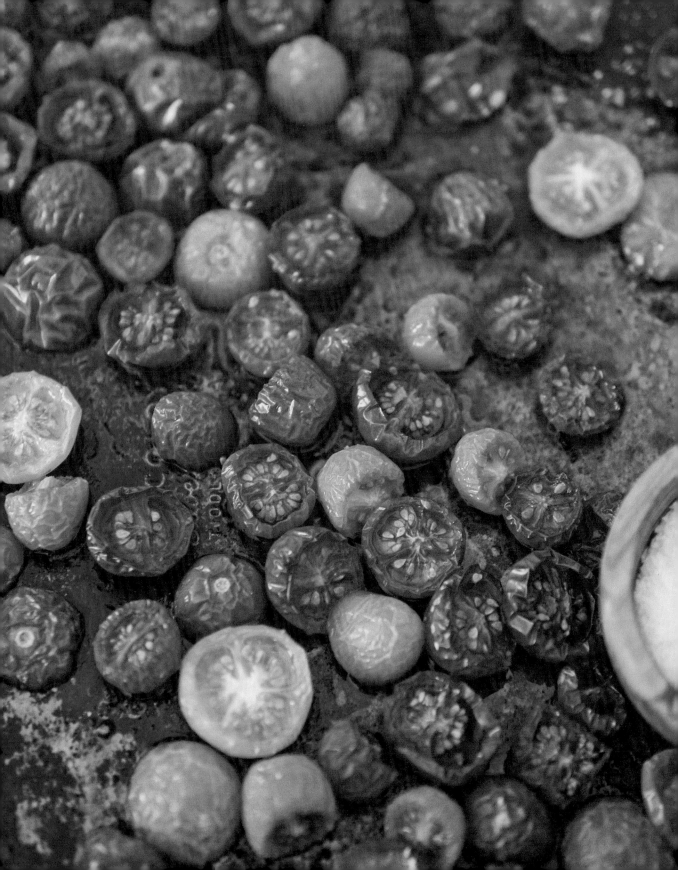

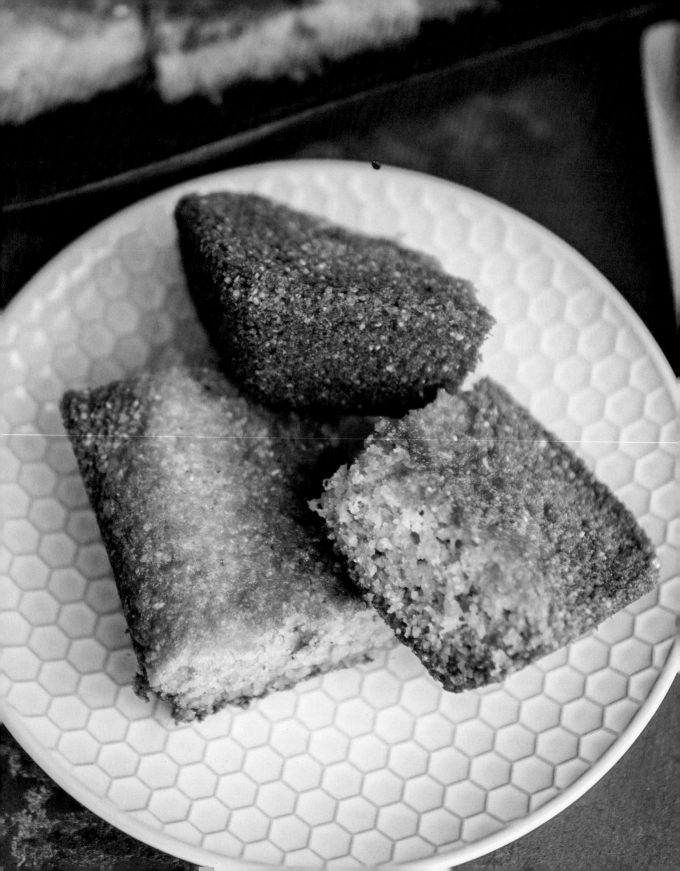

SWEET & MOIST CORN BREAD

SERVES: 10–12
PREP TIME: 10 MINUTES
COOK TIME: 35 MINUTES

1½ cups all-purpose flour

1 cup plus 2 tablespoons cornmeal

¾ teaspoon salt

¾ teaspoon baking soda

1 tablespoon baking powder

10 tablespoons butter, divided

6 tablespoons olive oil

1 cup granulated sugar

½ cup honey

3 large eggs

14 ounces buttermilk

THE FIRST bite of this corn bread will not only wake up your taste buds, but the slightly crisp outer crust paired with its soft and sweet inside crumb will keep you coming back for bite after bite. Whether it's one of those amazing attributes or a combination of them all, this Sweet & Moist Corn Bread is best baked in a screaming-hot cast-iron skillet for that perfect outer crust.

Preheat the oven to 375°F/190°C. Place a 12-inch cast-iron skillet in the oven as it preheats. Set the timer for 15 minutes to warm the skillet.

In a medium bowl, combine flour, cornmeal, salt, baking soda, and baking powder.

In a large bowl, add 8 tablespoons of butter. Melt the butter in the microwave in 15-second intervals. To the melted butter, add the olive oil, sugar, honey, eggs, and buttermilk. Mix until well combined. Pour the dry ingredients into the wet and mix with a silicone spatula until no large clumps remain.

When the timer sounds, remove the skillet from the oven and place 2 tablespoons of butter into the hot pan, spreading it out evenly to coat the bottom of the pan. Pour the corn bread batter into the hot skillet and place in the oven for 32–35 minutes until set and golden.

Allow the corn bread to cool for 15 minutes before slicing.

SIDES, SALADS & SANDWICHES

CHOURIÇO & CORN BREAD STUFFING

SERVES: 10–12
PREP TIME: 10 MINUTES
COOK TIME: 90 MINUTES

6 cups crusty bread, cubed

6 cups Sweet & Moist Corn Bread (see page 151 for recipe), cubed

1 tablespoon olive oil

½ pound chouriço, ground

1 cup white onion, diced

1 cup celery, diced

¼ cup parsley

½ teaspoon dried thyme

½ teaspoon dried rubbed sage

4 eggs, lightly beaten

5 cups low-sodium chicken broth

2 teaspoons salt

1 teaspoon black pepper

8 ounces pepper jack cheese, cubed

2 jalapeños, sliced

FOR THE last five years, this has been my contribution to our family Thanksgiving meal. It's a true collaboration with everyone bringing their special dish and, year after year, the meal remains pretty much the same. This stuffing quickly became a staple. Sweet corn bread, spicy chouriço, jalapeños, and cubes of pepper jack throughout. It's a hearty side, but Thanksgiving is all about that gobble-till-you-wobble approach.

Lay the crusty bread and corn bread cubes onto a large baking sheet. Allow the bread to sit out overnight to harden.

Preheat the oven to 350°F/177°C.

Heat a large skillet over medium heat and add the olive oil. When the oil shimmers, add the chouriço and cook, breaking it up into small bits, for 5–7 minutes. Add the onions and celery. Cover the skillet for 2 minutes to help sweat down the vegetables. Uncover and continue to cook until translucent and soft, about 3 minutes. Lastly, add the parsley, thyme, and sage. Remove the pan from the heat. In a large bowl, whisk the eggs, chicken broth, salt, and pepper.

In a 9x13 baking dish, mix the stale bread and corn bread. Add the chouriço, onions, celery, pepper jack cheese, and jalapeños. Pour the egg and broth mixture over the bread. Using two serving spoons or a spatula, toss to ensure everything is well incorporated and the breads are wet. Bake for 45 minutes.

Remove from the oven. Cool for 15 minutes before serving.

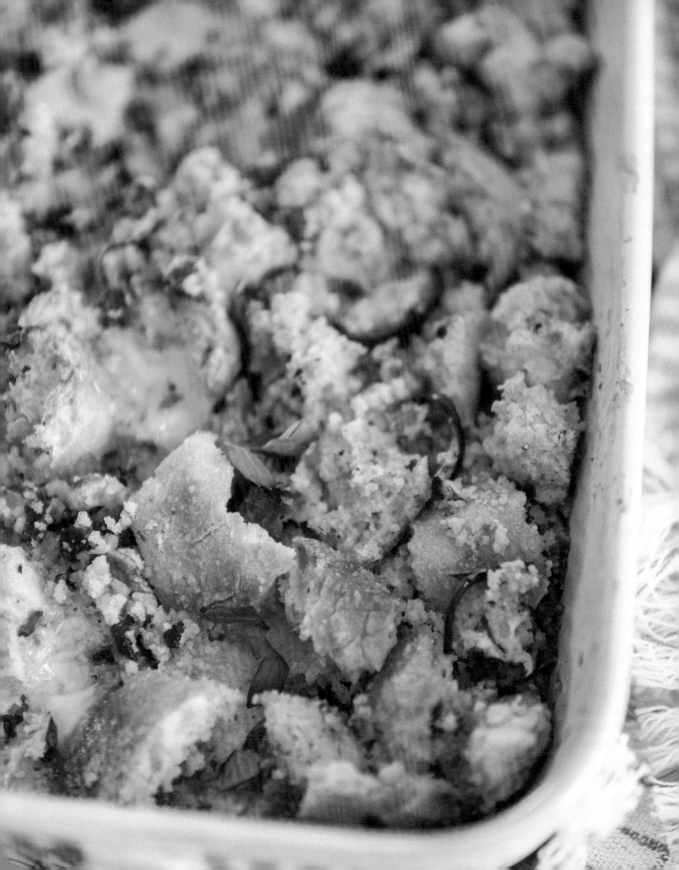

PERSIAN CUCUMBER CAPRESE

SERVES: 4
PREP TIME: 10 MINUTES
COOK TIME: 0 MINUTES

4 cups persian cucumbers, diced

2 cups mini heirloom tomatoes, halved

1–2 teaspoons salt to taste

¼ cup fresh basil leaves, torn

8 ounces mozzarella cheese pearls

1 tablespoon balsamic vinegar

2 tablespoons olive oil

Pinch red pepper flakes

PERSIAN CUCUMBERS are on my grocery list every week. They are fresh, crunchy, and a great addition to almost every meal. They can be simply prepared with a pinch of salt, rice vinegar, and sesame oil for an addition to Asian dishes or tossed with yogurt, dill, and za'atar seasoning for a quick tzatziki. Caprese is traditionally prepared with tomato and mozzarella. I'm starting a new caprese trend by making these crisp cucumbers the star ingredient.

In a large bowl, toss the cucumbers and tomatoes with 1–2 teaspoons of salt. Let sit for 2 minutes. Add the remaining ingredients and toss well to combine. Serve chilled.

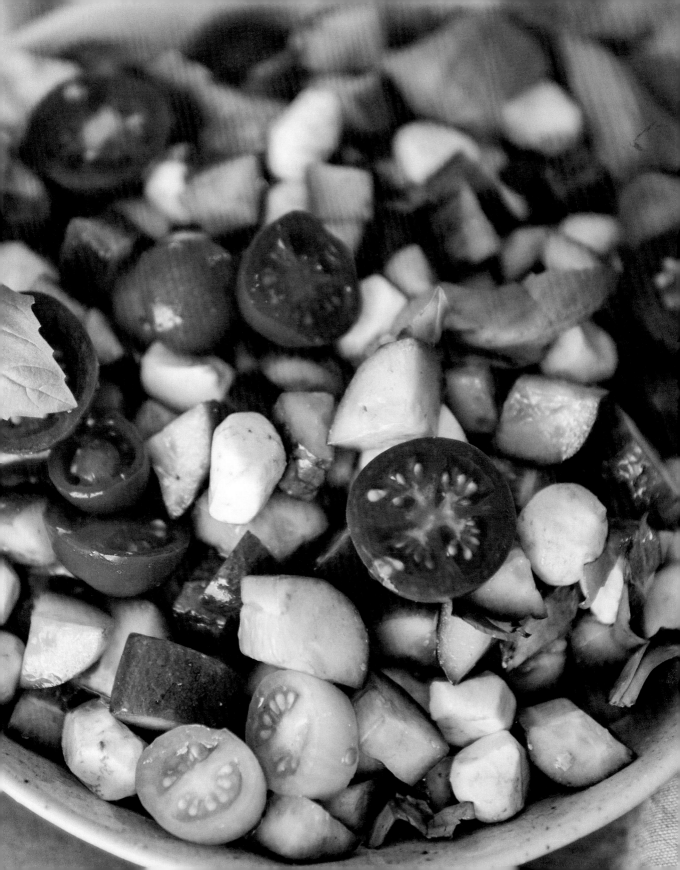

WATERMELON & AVOCADO SALAD

SERVES: 4
PREP TIME: 10 MINUTES
COOK TIME: 0 MINUTES

8 cups watermelon, diced

¼ cup red onion, minced

1 jalapeño, seeded and diced

2 tablespoons olive oil, divided

2 limes, juiced and divided

1 lime, zested

2 tablespoons honey

¼ teaspoon red pepper flakes

2 tablespoons fresh chives, chopped

1 cup fresh basil, torn

4 ounces feta cheese, crumbled

3–4 ripe avocados

Kosher salt

SOMETHING ABOUT this combination works in a way I would not have assumed. When I think of watermelon, the only food memories that come to mind are juicy slices on a hot summer day. Creating recipes for this book helped push my imagination. Now, pairing jalapeños, basil, and feta with watermelon doesn't seem so crazy.

To a large bowl, add the diced watermelon, red onion, and jalapeño. In a small bowl, whisk 1 tablespoon of olive oil, juice of 1 lime, lime zest, honey, and red pepper flakes. Pour the dressing over the watermelon and toss to coat. To the dressed watermelon, add the chives, basil, and feta. Toss and set aside.

Add the avocado to the bowl of a food processor with the remaining tablespoon of olive oil and lime juice. Add a generous pinch of salt and process until smooth, about 1 minute. To serve, spread the avocado puree on the bottom of your serving platter or evenly spread onto each plate. Top the avocado puree with the dressed watermelon. Serve chilled.

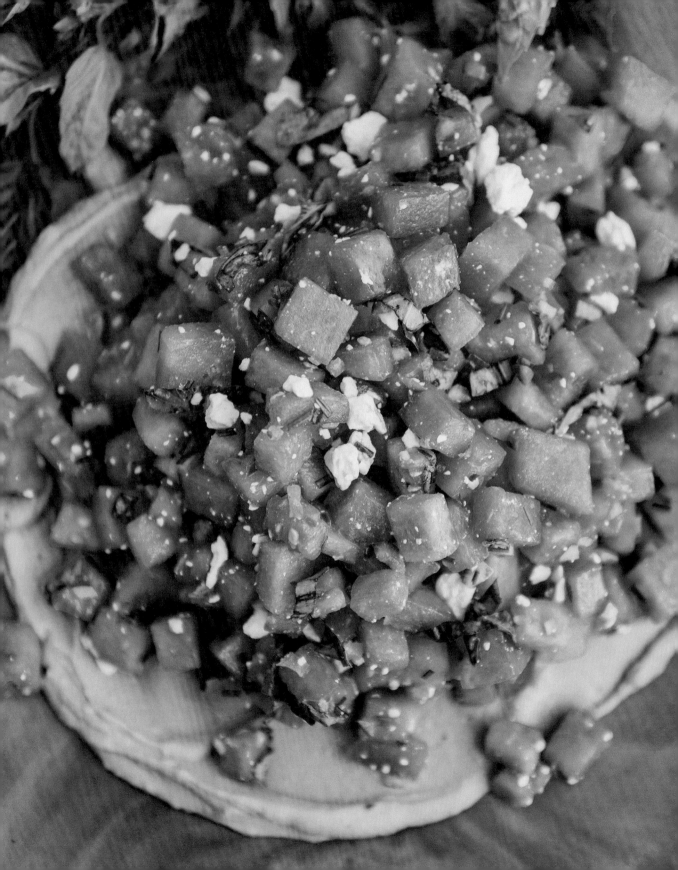

GRILLED CORN & CUCUMBER SALAD

SERVES: 4
PREP TIME: 10 MINUTES
COOK TIME: 20 MINUTES

2 ears sweet corn, husked
1 tablespoon olive oil
Salt and pepper to taste
2 Persian cucumbers, cubed
1 ripe avocado, diced
3 scallions, diced
2 tablespoons lime juice
½ cup cilantro leaves

WITH THE travel we've done over the years to various cities and countries for competitions during Mat's career, we've always tried to bring some comforts of home with us. Whether that be traveling with a pillow or a favorite coffee or finding a place with a kitchen or kitchenette, I created this recipe in a hotel in London, England. Mat was competing and I was trying to make the most of a very small kitchen in a different country. Believe it or not, the original toss-together recipe used frozen corn quick cooked on a small stove top. It packed great crunch and familiar flavors and remains a side dish we re-create often.

Preheat the grill to 400°F/200°C. Coat the ears of corn with olive oil and season with salt and pepper. When the grill is hot, roast the corn for 15–20 minutes until the kernels are cooked and the corn is slightly charred. Allow the corn to cool on a cutting board for 10 minutes before handling.

While the corn cooks, prepare the other ingredients. In a large bowl, toss the cubed cucumbers with a pinch of salt. Add the diced avocado, scallions, and lime juice. When the corn is cooled enough to handle, stand it on its end and cut the kernels away from the cob. Add the cut corn to the bowl and toss to combine. Taste and add salt as needed. Finish by adding the cilantro leaves and toss once more. Serve immediately (with Spiced Chicken with Green Sauce on page 64) or cover and refrigerate for future use.

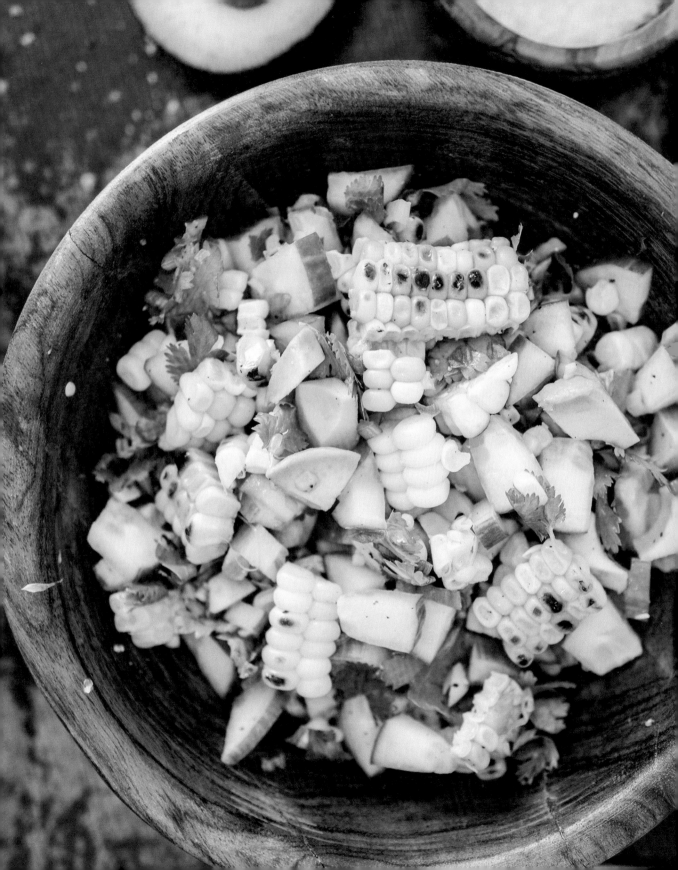

GRILLED STONE FRUIT & HONEY-BASIL SALAD

SERVES: 4
PREP TIME: 10 MINUTES
COOK TIME: 25 MINUTES

2 peaches, thick sliced

2 nectarines, thick sliced

2 plums, thick sliced

½ cup and 2 tablespoons olive oil, divided

2 ears sweet corn, husked

1 cup fresh basil

1 tablespoon honey

1 tablespoon whole-grain dijon mustard

¼ cup rice vinegar

Pinch flaky salt

1 cup arugula

3 cups spring mix lettuce

¼ cup radish, thin sliced

4 (2-ounce) burrata balls, quartered

SUMMER IS my favorite time of the year for fresh fruits and sweet summer corn. These fruits pair perfectly with strong herbs like basil and balance the pepperiness of arugula. Combine all that with oozy burrata cheese and you have yourself a winning summer dish. Easily learn the seasons by visiting your local farmers' market to collect available ingredients and cook a seasonal dish like this one.

Preheat the grill (or a grill pan) to 350–400°F/177–200°C (or over medium heat). In a medium bowl, toss the peaches, nectarines, and plums with 1 tablespoon of olive oil. Set aside.

Drizzle the corn with one tablespoon of olive oil and work with your hands to fully coat. Place the corn directly on the grill for 15 minutes, flipping once or twice throughout the cook until lightly charred.

Add the mixed stone fruit to the grill directly onto the grates grill for 10 minutes, flipping halfway.

Place the basil, honey, mustard, and rice vinegar into the bowl of a food processor. Blitz for 1 minute. While the processor is running, pour the ½ cup of olive oil into the food chute. Taste and add a pinch of salt as needed. Set aside.

Remove the fruit and corn from the grill. Cool for 5 minutes before handling. Cut the corn kernels off the cob, taste and add a pinch of flaky salt as needed.

To assemble the salad, toss the arugula and spring mix in a large bowl. Add the radish and corn, toss again. Top the salad with the grilled fruit slices and burrata. Dress with 2–4 tablespoons of honey-basil dressing.

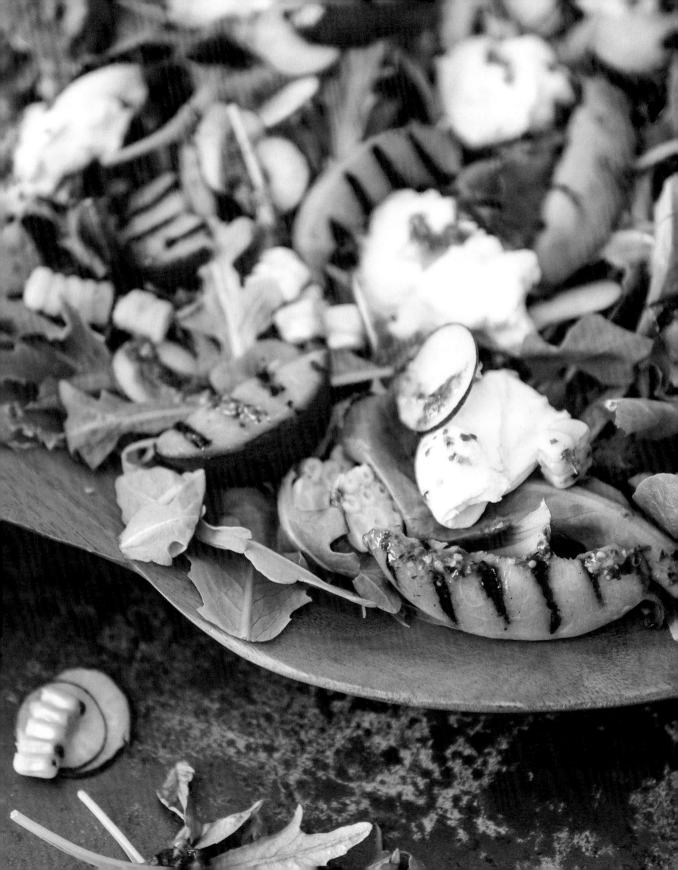

KALE & HAZELNUT SALAD WITH SHERRY-SHALLOT VINAIGRETTE

SERVES: 4
PREP TIME: 15 MINUTES
COOK TIME: 0 MINUTES

2 bunches Tuscan/dino kale, de-stemmed and roughly chopped

1 tablespoon lemon juice

Pinch salt

½ cup celery, thinly sliced

1 cup red grapes, halved

¼ cup roasted hazelnuts

2–4 tablespoons Sherry Shallot Vinaigrette

1 ripe avocado, diced

Freshly grated Parmesan cheese for serving

THE STAR of this salad is the hazelnuts. Normally, I'd recommend swapping ingredients as needed for what you have on hand, but in this case, hunt down the hazelnuts in the store. It's a rather unique ingredient, but I've also used them in a couple of recipes in this book to make it worth your investment (see page 52 for Hickory-Smoked Pecan Granola recipe, or see page 198 for Pretzel, Hazelnut & Peanut Butter Icebox Cake recipe).

To start, de-stem the kale by holding the stem in one hand and placing three fingers of your other hand at the base of the leaves. Pull your fingers along the stem, tearing the leaves off. Lay your leaves on your cutting board and cut across the leaf into slices. Into a large serving bowl, mix the sliced kale, lemon juice, and a good pinch of salt. Massage the kale for 1–2 minutes between your hands to soften slightly. Add the thinly sliced celery and red grapes. Toss to combine.

Place the hazelnuts in a small plastic bag. Using a meat tenderizer (a measuring cup or mason jar would work too!), smash the hazelnuts slightly to break them up. Add the hazelnuts to the kale, toss to combine. Dress the salad with 2–4 tablespoons of Sherry Shallot Vinaigrette (see opposite for recipe). Toss well, taste, and salt as needed or add additional dressing to your preference. Lastly, add the diced avocado. Toss gently once or twice and serve with freshly grated Parmesan.

FEEDING THE FRASERS

162

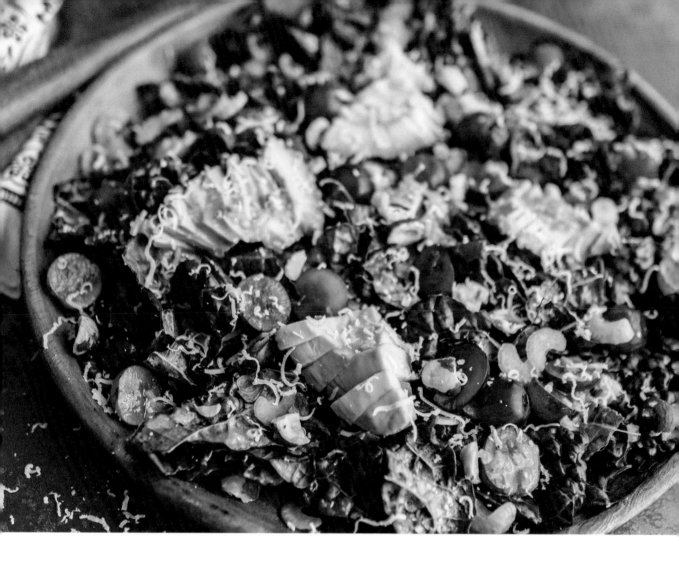

SHERRY-SHALLOT VINAIGRETTE

YIELDS: *1 CUP*
PREP TIME: *10 MINUTES*
COOK TIME: *0 MINUTES*

¼ cup sherry vinegar

2 teaspoons dijon mustard

1 teaspoon kosher salt

Pinch fresh ground black pepper

¼ cup finely minced shallots

⅔ cup olive oil

In a small mixing bowl, whisk the sherry vinegar, dijon mustard, salt, and pepper to taste. Stir in the shallots. Gradually whisk in the oil to create a smooth dressing. Use immediately or store in a mason jar in the refrigerator.

GARLIC-GRILLED CHICKEN CHOP

SERVES: 4

PREP TIME: 15 MINUTES

COOK TIME: 45 MINUTES

1 pound carrots, cut into 1 inch slices

2 tablespoons olive oil

1 teaspoon salt

½ teaspoon pepper

4 chicken breasts

Salt and pepper to taste

1 tablespoon garlic powder

2 teaspoons onion powder

2 teaspoons dried parsley

½ teaspoon dried dill

Pinch red pepper flakes

Flaky sea salt to taste

4 cups romaine lettuce, chopped

2 tablespoons fresh dill

2 tablespoons fresh parsley

2 cups english cucumber, diced

1 cup red grapes, halved

4 ounces feta cheese crumbles

1 ripe avocado, quartered and sliced

SOME OF my favorite salad creations came to be by emptying the fridge of random fresh and roasted vegetables, cooked proteins, and whatever leafy greens sat in the crisper. If I'm being completely honest, these creations were mainly to unload the ends of these containers to make room for the next round of cooked meals—an everything-but-the-kitchen-sink mentality. If it looks like it's on its last day in the fridge before it meets the trash bin, let's add it to a salad! I'm sure I'm not the only one out there with this approach! This recipe is now one I intentionally make after grabbing the odds and ends from the fridge that one day.

Preheat the oven to 400°F/200°C. In a large bowl, toss the carrots with olive oil, salt, and pepper to evenly coat. Spread the carrots out in one layer on a baking sheet. To allow plenty of space for crisping, use two baking sheets if needed. Roast for 15–20 minutes. Toss and roast an additional 10–25 minutes until fork tender and golden brown.

While the carrots are roasting, preheat the grill to 375°F/190°C. Season the chicken breasts with salt and pepper. In a small bowl, mix the garlic powder, onion powder, parsley, dill, and red pepper flakes. Toss seasoning with the chicken to fully coat. Grill the chicken for 7–10 minutes on one side. Flip and continue cooking for an additional 7–10 minutes or until the internal temperature reaches 165°F/73°C.

Remove the chicken from the grill and rest for 5 minutes before slicing. While the chicken rests, prepare the remaining ingredients for the salad.

Remove the carrots from the oven, sprinkle with flaky sea salt to taste.

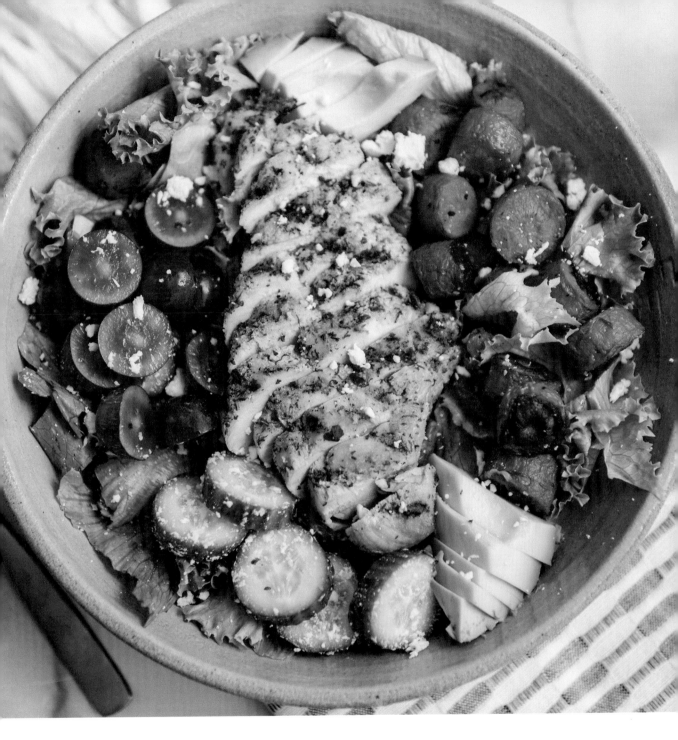

In a large salad bowl, toss the chopped romaine lettuce, fresh dill, and fresh parsley.
Top the lettuce mix with the English cucumbers, red grapes, and feta cheese. Add the
roasted carrots and avocado. Top with sliced chicken and serve.

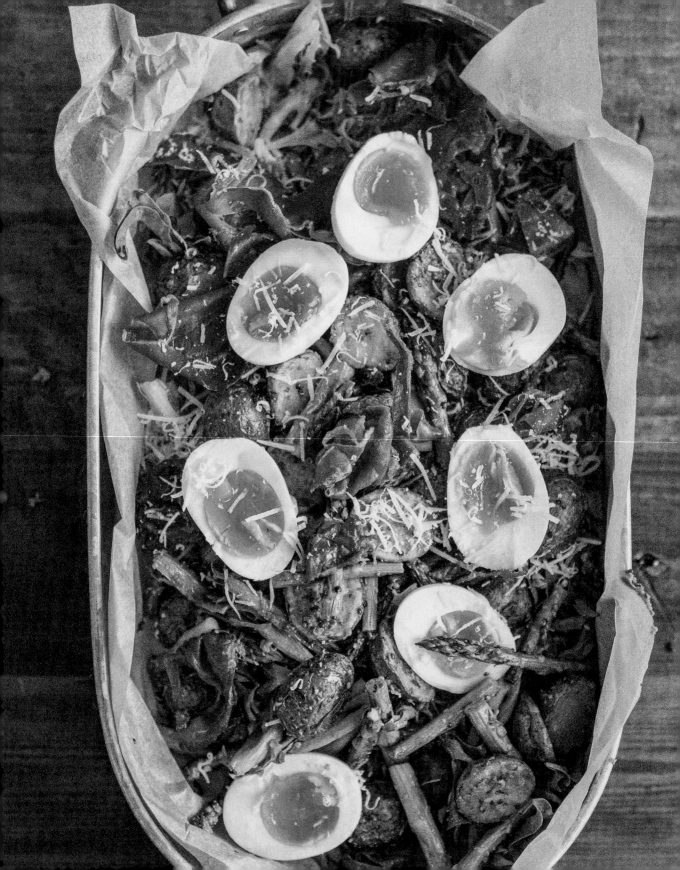

HERBY GREENS, ROASTED POTATOES & SEVEN-MINUTE EGG SALAD

SERVES: 4

PREP TIME: 10 MINUTES

COOK TIME: 15 MINUTES

Mustard-Roasted Potatoes & Asparagus (see page 144 for recipe)

4 ounces prosciutto

12 ounces spring mix lettuce or baby kale

¼ fresh parsley leaves

2 tablespoons fresh dill

¼ cup fresh radish, diced

8 Seven-Minute Eggs (see page 2 for recipe), halved

¼ cup grated Parmesan cheese

I ABSOLUTELY love mixing fresh herbs into my salad greens. One of the local farmers' market vendors sells a bag of mixed greens, and she always adds the most unlikely herbs to the bunch. It brings an element of surprise to each bag. Ever since my first salad with her mixed greens, I've been adding a pop of fresh herbs to my salads.

Preheat the Traeger Grill (or conventional grill or oven) to 400°F/200°C. While the potatoes are roasting, cook the prosciutto by curling strips of prosciutto on a separate ¼ baking sheet. Bake in the Traeger for 15 minutes or until desired doneness. Remove the prosciutto from the grill and set aside.

In a large salad bowl, toss the spring mix, parsley leaves, dill, and radish. Top the salad with the Mustard-Roasted Potatoes & Asparagus, crispy prosciutto, and Seven-Minute Eggs. Sprinkle with grated Parmesan cheese and serve.

BLACKBERRY, PROSCIUTTO & BRIE TARTINE

SERVES: 4
PREP TIME: 10 MINUTES
COOK TIME: 45 MINUTES

4 slices sourdough bread, toasted and cut in half

½ cup Blackberry-Chia Jam (see recipe on page 54)

8 ounces brie, cut into long slices (with rind)

8 ounces prosciutto, torn

TARTINE IS the fancy word for an open-faced sandwich, and if we're calling a spade a spade, it's toast! This is a cheese board smeared atop a crispy slice of sourdough. I love having a cheese board for nibbling while entertaining friends or during holiday family gatherings, and this is a great way to use up those cheese board leftovers (if there are any!) or just a tasty sweet and savory bite.

Preheat the oven to high broil.

On a baking sheet, lay the cuts of toasted bread. Spread each slice with Blackberry-Chia Jam. Top the jam with slices of brie and torn pieces of prosciutto.

Place the baking sheet on the top shelf in the oven under the broiler. Broil for 3–5 minutes until the brie begins to melt. Watch carefully as to not burn the tartine. Remove from the oven and serve immediately.

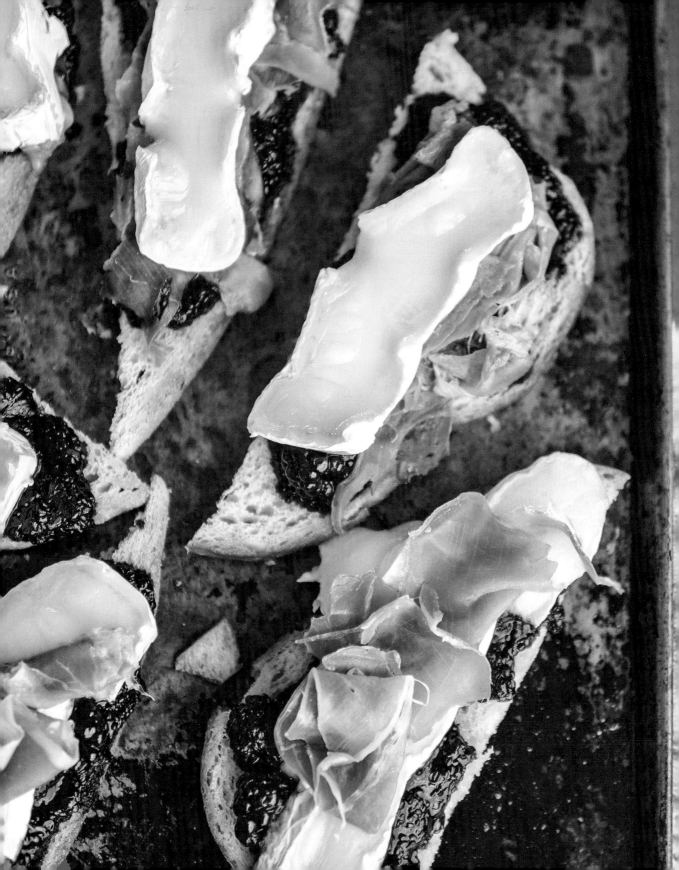

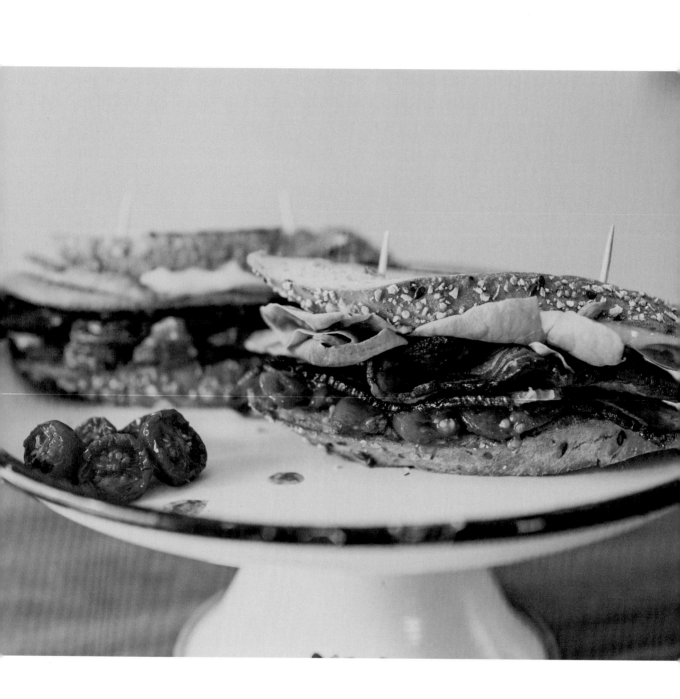

SMOKY BLT

SERVES: 4
PREP TIME: 10 MINUTES
COOK TIME: 20 MINUTES

8 slices of thick-cut bacon

1 teaspoon cracked black pepper

½ teaspoon cayenne pepper

½ teaspoon smoked paprika

Smoked Tomatoes (see page 148 for recipe)

Multigrain baguette, sliced and toasted

Iceberg lettuce

4 tablespoons mayonnaise

WHEN I first started writing recipes for this book, I'd ask friends and family this question: "When you order at a restaurant, what is your go-to? The answers were insightful. The most consistent answer was a BLT. If I'm serving a BLT, it's not going to be just your average, everyday BLT. We have put some serious flavor into a very simple sandwich.

Preheat the oven to 350°F/177°C. Line a baking sheet with aluminum foil. Lay the strips of bacon on the aluminum foil–lined baking sheet and sprinkle with the cracked black pepper, cayenne, and smoked paprika. Toss with your hands to evenly coat the bacon, redistribute on the tray, and bake for 15–20 minutes until the bacon is crisp. Remove the bacon from the oven and lay on a paper towel–lined plate.

To assemble the sandwich, smear 1–2 tablespoons of smoked tomatoes on one slice of toasted bread. Top the tomatoes with 2 slices of bacon. Add a layer or two of lettuce and close the sandwich with an additional piece of toasted bread smeared with mayonnaise.

SIDES, SALADS & SANDWICHES

TURKEY-AVOCADO SAMMICH

SERVES: 4
PREP TIME: 15 MINUTES
COOK TIME: 20 MINUTES

8 slices thick-cut bacon

8 slices sourdough sandwich bread, toasted

4–8 tablespoons mayonnaise

2 pounds oven-roasted turkey breast, deli sliced

1 ripe avocado, sliced

¼ cup sprouts

1 large tomato, sliced

4 slices cheddar or colby jack cheese

I HAVE to credit all my love for this sandwich to the Well-Fed Fraser. He is the sandwich guru. I spent years making him turkey sandwiches, never to sit and enjoy one myself. I was convinced I didn't like sandwiches. Let me tell you, I was wrong! Turns out, I *love* sandwiches and specifically this one here. I eat this sandwich (or a variation of it) daily. I hope you find the same joy sandwiches have brought to my daily food lineup with this Turkey-Avocado Sammich.

Preheat the oven to 350°F/177°C. Lay the strips of bacon onto an aluminum foil-lined baking sheet. Bake for 15–20 minutes or until desired doneness. Move the bacon to a paper towel–lined plate and set aside.

To assemble the sandwich, spread each slice of toasted bread with mayonnaise. Evenly distribute the turkey slices among the four sandwiches. To the turkey, add 2 slices of bacon, sliced avocado, 2 tablespoons of sprouts, 1–2 slices of tomato, and a slice of cheese. Top each sandwich with the remaining slice of bread, cut the sandwich in half, and enjoy!

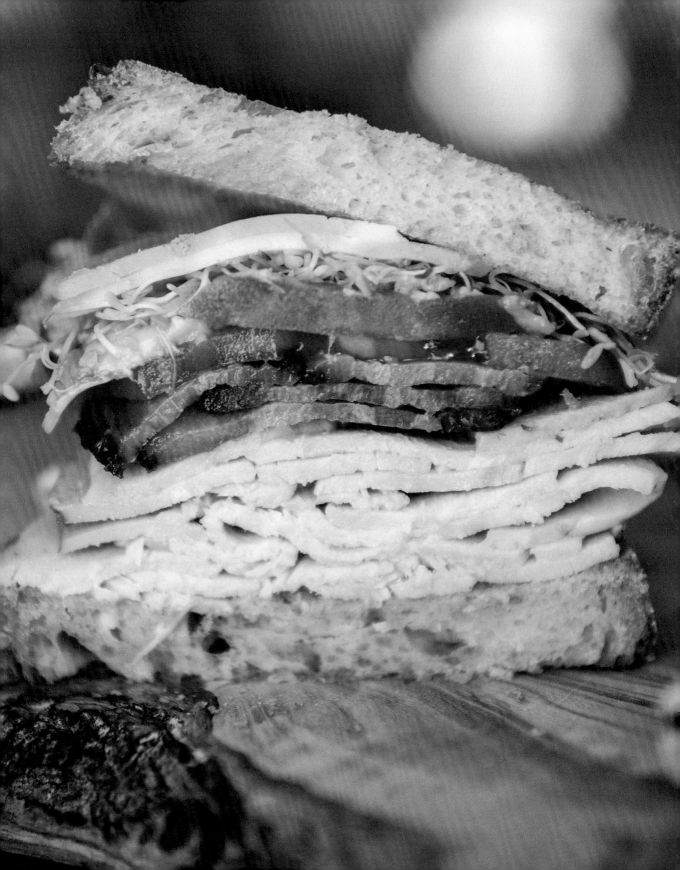

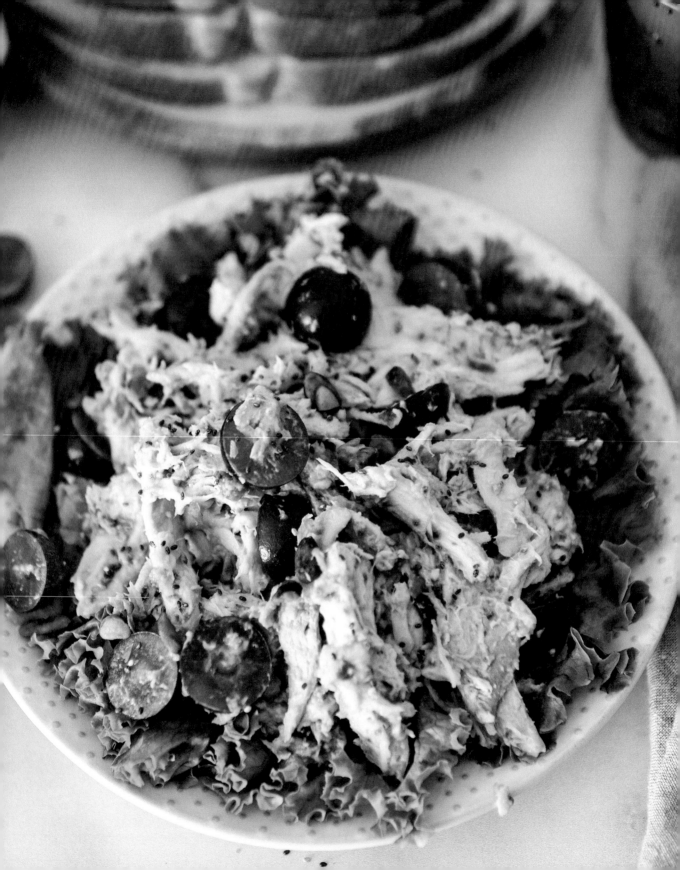

MAPLE MUSTARD CHICKEN SALAD

SERVES: 6–8
PREP TIME: 15 MINUTES
COOK TIME: 0 MINUTES

4 cups leftover Spatchcock Chicken (see page 62 for recipe), shredded

¼ cup roasted pistachios, chopped

1 cup red grapes, halved

2 ripe avocados, mashed

2 tablespoons mayonnaise

1 tablespoon maple syrup

1 tablespoon dijon mustard

2 teaspoons chia seeds

Salt and pepper to taste

CHICKEN SALAD is a weekly staple in our house. Anytime I have the chance to tuck leftovers into a new dish, I'm IN! Not to mention the pop of fresh grapes and the crunch of roasted nuts make each bite fresh and exciting. Feel free to get creative with your add-ins. The below are our favorites, but you can swap the grapes for dried cranberries or pomegranate arils and substitute the pistachios for roasted almonds or pecans. You get to be the boss in your own kitchen!

In a large bowl, combine the shredded chicken, pistachios, and red grapes.

In a separate medium bowl, mix the mashed avocado, mayonnaise, maple syrup, dijon mustard, and chia seeds.

Add the dressing to the large bowl of chicken. Toss to combine. Taste and season with salt and pepper as needed.

Serve on a bed of greens, in a wrap, or between two slices of toasted bread.

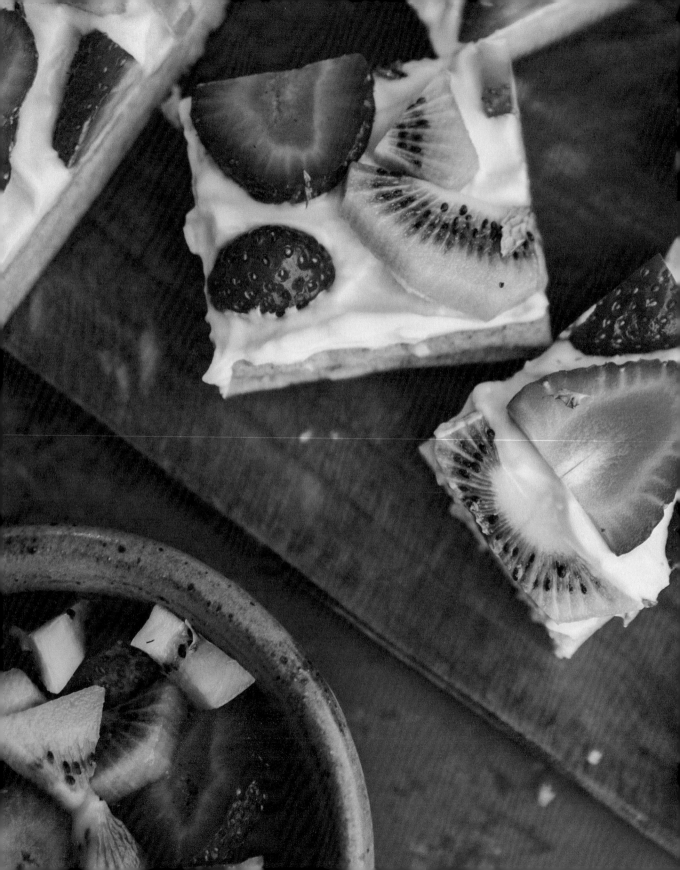

SNACKS & SWEETS

MEXICAN STREET CORN GUACAMOLE

YIELDS: 4 CUPS
PREP TIME: 10 MINUTES
COOK TIME: 25 MINUTES

2 ears corn, husked

½ tablespoon olive oil

Salt and pepper to taste

4 ripe avocados

Juice of 1 lime

¼ cup red onion, diced

1 jalapeño, diced

½ cup cilantro leaves

½ cup cotija cheese, divided

1 teaspoon lime zest

1 teaspoon chili powder

Salt to taste

Pinch of ancho chili powder

THIS MEXICAN Street Corn Guacamole combines my two favorite side dishes with smooth and creamy ripe avocados and the pop and crunch of grilled corn. It's all pulled together with salty cotija cheese and a hit of spice from the chili. My mouth is watering just describing it! I could happily sit down with a bowl of this and a bag of perfectly salted tortilla chips and be set for the night.

Preheat the grill to 450–500°F/230–260°C. Drizzle the corn with olive oil and season with salt and pepper. Place the corn directly on the grill grates and grill for 5–7 minutes per side until cooked and charred.

In a medium bowl, mix the ripe avocado, lime juice, red onion, jalapeño, and cilantro leaves until well combined. Set aside.

Remove the corn from the grill and cool for 5–10 minutes until cool enough to handle. Using a sharp knife, remove the charred kernels from the cob and place in a medium bowl. Add ¼ cup of cotija cheese, lime zest, and chili powder until well incorporated.

To the bowl of avocados, mix all but ¼ cup of corn. Taste and season with salt as needed. Top the guacamole with the remaining corn and cotija cheese, sprinkle with ancho chili powder, and serve with corn tortilla chips.

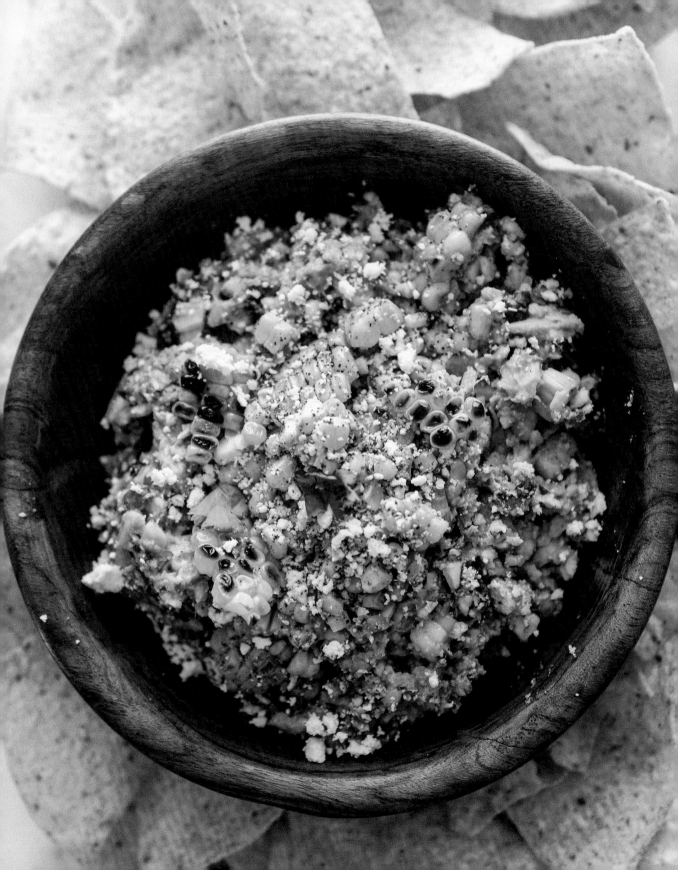

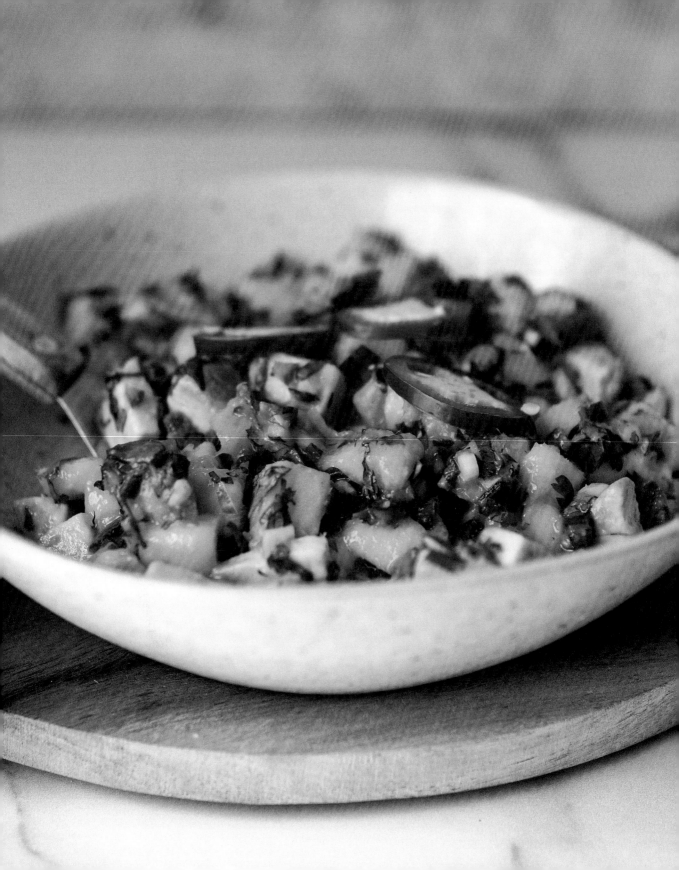

JALAPEÑO-MINT-MANGO SALSA

SERVES: 4–6
PREP TIME: 10 MINUTES
COOK TIME: 0 MINUTES

3 mangos, diced

1 whole jalapeño, diced

¼ cup red onion, diced

1 avocado, diced

1 lime, juiced

½ cup cilantro leaves and stems, finely chopped

2 teaspoons fresh mint, finely chopped

Flaky salt to taste

FRESH, SPICY, and slightly sweet, this makes for a great appetizer served with perfectly salted tortilla chips or a fresh addition to grilled meats for dinner. Top your latest taco creations with a scoop or two of this zingy salsa or serve it with Blackened Mahi Mahi (see page 114 for recipe).

In a medium mixing bowl, toss the ingredients until well combined. Taste and add a generous pinch of flaky salt. Taste and adjust salt as needed.

Cover and chill until ready to use. Serve atop grilled chicken or fish or with a side of tortilla chips.

SMOKED GARLIC & ZA'ATAR HUMMUS

YIELDS: 3½ CUPS
PREP TIME: 5 MINUTES
COOK TIME: 0 MINUTES

¼ cup tahini

2 tablespoons lemon juice

10 smoked/roasted garlic cloves, roughly chopped

2 (15-ounce) cans garbanzo beans, drained and rinsed (⅓ cup liquid reserved)

1 teaspoon za'atar, plus more for serving

1 teaspoon salt, plus more to taste

3 tablespoons olive oil, plus more for serving

I CANNOT believe I spent so many years buying hummus at the local stores. Smooth and creamy, rich in flavor, and loaded with simple ingredients, hummus is a staple in our house, easy for entertaining, and a great addition to many meals. Spread hummus on a burger bun, or scoop a dollop into a chopped salad for added flavor and richness.

In a food processor, place tahini and lemon juice. Blitz for 1 minute until pale and slightly fluffy. Scrape down the sides and the bottom of the bowl, blitz for an additional 30 seconds to 1 minute.

With the food processor running, add the smoked/roasted garlic to the food chute. Run the food processor for 30 seconds for the garlic to fully incorporate. Turn the food processor off, add ½ of the garbanzo beans and garbanzo bean liquid. Blitz for 1 minute, scrape down the sides and bottom of the bowl, and add the remaining beans. Turn the processor on for an additional 2 minutes, scraping down halfway.

Add the za'atar and salt, then with the food processor running, add 3 tablespoons of olive oil and blend an additional 30 seconds to 1 minute until incorporated and smooth. Taste and adjust salt as needed, running the food processor again to blend if you've added more.

Move the hummus to a serving dish, garnish with a heavy pour of olive oil, and sprinkle with a pinch or two of za'atar. Serve with fresh vegetables like cucumber slices, carrots, and pita chips.

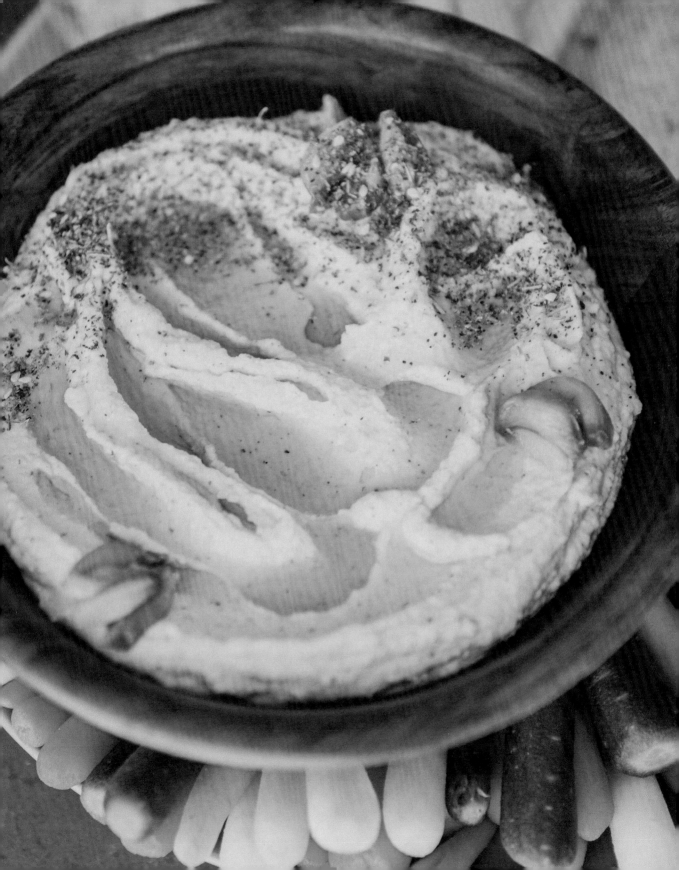

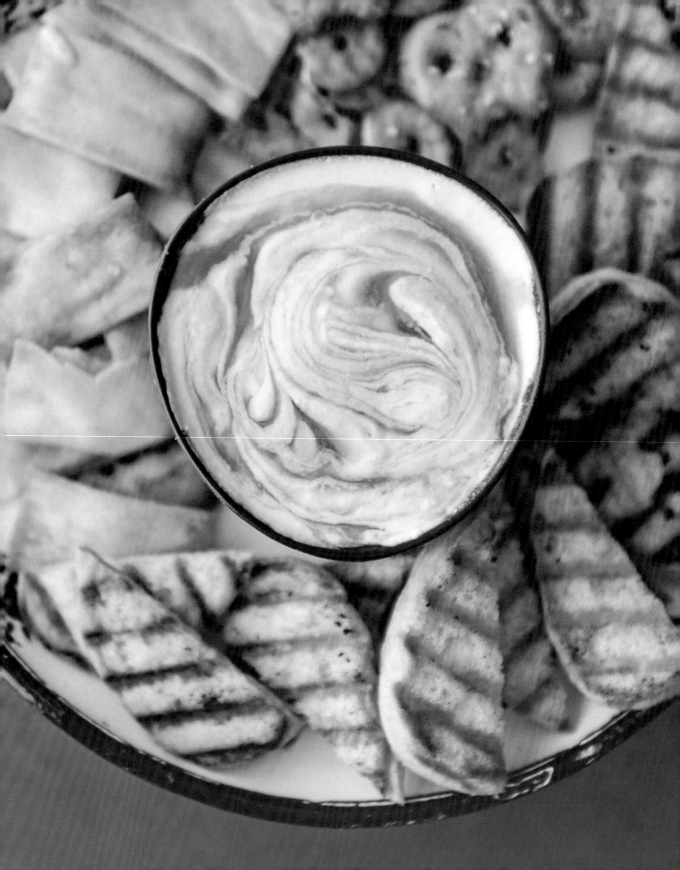

SWEET & SPICY WHIPPED CHEESE

SERVES: 6
PREP TIME: 5 MINUTES
COOK TIME: 0 MINUTES

4 ounces feta

4 ounces goat cheese

2 ounces plain greek yogurt

2 tablespoons Hot Honey
(recipe below)

THIS RICH and creamy dip satisfies all the salty-sweet cravings. It's best made with room-temperature ingredients to get a smooth whip and can be chilled before serving. Leftover whipped cheese (without Hot Honey) can be used for Whipped Feta & Egg Toastie (see page 10 for recipe).

Place all ingredients in the bowl of a stand mixer with the whisk attachment. You may also use a large bowl with an electric handheld mixer. Whip until smooth, about 2 minutes. Spoon into serving dish and top with a drizzle of Hot Honey. Serve with pita chips or crispy grilled bread.

HOT HONEY

YIELDS ABOUT ½ CUP
PREP TIME: 5 MINUTES
COOK TIME: 0 MINUTES

¼ cup honey

4 tablespoons butter, melted

2 teaspoons cayenne pepper

½ teaspoon chili powder

½ teaspoon smoked paprika

1 tablespoon apple cider vinegar

Pinch salt

In a small bowl, whisk all the ingredients until fully combined. Store in a mason jar in the refrigerator and reheat in the microwave in increments to soften when ready to use again.

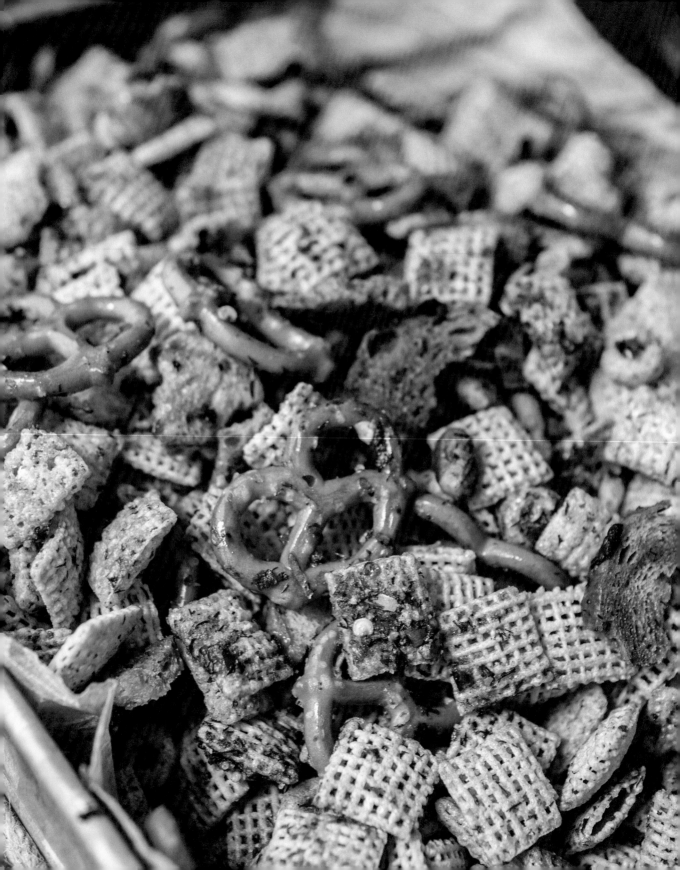

FIERY RANCH CHEX MIX

YIELDS: 12 CUPS
PREP TIME: 10 MINUTES
COOK TIME: 25 MINUTES

½ cup salted butter, melted

¼ cup olive oil

2 tablespoons honey

2 tablespoons red pepper flakes

1 tablespoon dried parsley

5 teaspoons dried dill

2 teaspoons onion powder

2 teaspoons dried minced onion

2 teaspoons onion salt

1½ teaspoons garlic powder

1 teaspoon smoked paprika

1 teaspoon ancho chili powder

3 cups Rice Chex

4 cups Corn Chex

2 cups pretzels

1 cup bagel chips (from leftover Onion Bagels)

1 cup plain Cheerios

1 cup roasted pistachios

WE ARE not big-time snackers. Snacks really only come out when there's a swarm of friends or family around the kitchen island. Something about swapping stories and nibbling on something spicy just works!

Preheat the oven to 300°F/150°C.

In a medium bowl, combine the melted butter and oil. To the butter and oil, add the honey and all the spice ingredients and mix into a paste. In a large mixing bowl, toss the remaining ingredients.

Pour the spice butter mixture over the dry ingredients. Toss until well incorporated and fully coated. Evenly distribute the mixture onto an aluminum foil- or parchment paper–lined baking sheet.

Bake for 25 minutes, tossing once or twice throughout the cook time. Remove from the oven and cool completely. Store in an airtight container on the counter for 3–5 days (if it lasts that long!).

PRO TIP

Turn your Onion Bagel (see page 20 for recipe) into the bagel chips used in this recipe. A much better alternative to store-bought and also a great way to transform one recipe into another. Simply slice the bagels thin, toss with olive oil, and bake at 350°F/177°C for 10 minutes until browned and crispy.

CHURRO CHEERIO CHEX MIX

YIELDS: 12 CUPS
PREP TIME: 20 MINUTES
COOK TIME: 40 MINUTES

1 cup butter, melted and divided

½ cup brown sugar

1 tablespoon cinnamon, divided

1½ teaspoons vanilla extract, divided

2 cups oyster crackers

2 cups plain Cheerios

2 tablespoons granulated sugar

Pinch kosher salt

½ cup honey

2 cups Rice Chex

2 cups Corn Chex

2 cups Teddy Grahams

1 cup sliced almonds

IT'S EASY to spot the true sweet snackers with this Churro Cheerio Chex Mix. It doesn't last long in our house and makes for a great treat when entertaining. We typically make this and the Fiery Ranch Chex Mix (see page 187 for recipe) at the same time. You can bounce from bowl to bowl. A few handfuls of savory and spicy and then a few handfuls of sweet!

Preheat the oven to 300°F/150°C.

In a large mixing bowl, whisk ½ cup of melted butter, brown sugar, 1 teaspoon of cinnamon, and ½ teaspoon of vanilla extract. Add the oyster crackers and plain Cheerios, toss to fully incorporate. Spread the mix onto a parchment-lined baking sheet. Bake for 10–12 minutes until bubbly. Meanwhile, in a small bowl, mix the granulated sugar, the remaining 2 teaspoons of cinnamon, and salt, set aside.

In a separate large mixing bowl, whisk the remaining ½ cup of melted butter, honey, and 1 teaspoon of vanilla extract. To the bowl, add the Chex, Teddy Grahams, and almonds. Mix until fully coated. Spread the mixture evenly onto another parchment-lined baking sheet. Bake for 25 minutes, tossing once or twice throughout the bake.

When the oyster crackers and Cheerios have finished baking, remove them from the oven and sprinkle with the cinnamon-sugar mix. Allow it to completely cool, about 15 minutes. Once it's completely cooled, break it into small pieces. Set the churro Cheerio mix aside.

Remove the Chex from the oven, top with the churro Cheerios mix, and cool completely. Once the mix has cooled, toss to fully combine and break into small pieces. Store in an airtight container on the counter for 3–5 days (if it lasts that long!).

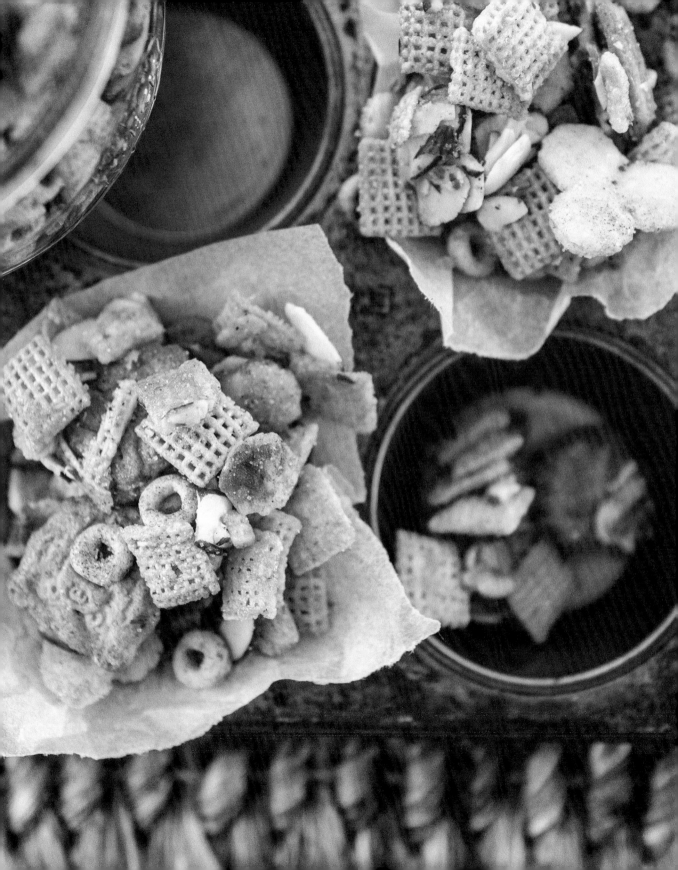

COCONUT SWEET RICE

SERVES: *8–10*

PREP TIME: *10 MINUTES*

COOK TIME: *40 MINUTES*

1 cup jasmine rice

¼ teaspoon salt

2 cups water

1 cinnamon stick

1 lemon rind

2 cups hot canned coconut milk (just liquid, not the cream at the top)

½ cup granulated sugar

¼ cup brown sugar

1 tablespoon salted butter

1 teaspoon vanilla extract

2 egg yolks

Ground cinnamon for garnish

I GREW up in a predominantly Portuguese part of town. Almost all my childhood friends spoke Portuguese as their first language, and it was the primary language at home. I didn't go to many arcade or roller rink birthday parties. The middle school and high school family gatherings or friends' birthday parties were in a stacked house with their large extended families sitting on plastic-lined couches and potluck meals of caçoila and bacalhau. Cake and ice cream were always served at these parties, but I knew someone's *vovó* (grandmother) had made a batch of sweet rice.

In a medium saucepan, bring the rice, salt, and water to a boil. Reduce the heat, add the cinnamon stick and lemon rind. Cook stirring occasionally for 10–15 minutes until most of the water is absorbed.

Heat the coconut milk in the microwave until hot but not boiling. Stir in the sugars, butter, and vanilla. Temper the egg yolks by spooning ¼ cup of the hot coconut milk mixture into a small bowl with the yolks and whisk. This will help ensure that the yolks do not turn into scrambled eggs when added to the hot rice. Mix the yolks in with the coconut milk mixture. Lastly, add everything to the cooking rice. Stir and cover.

Simmer on low for 15–20 minutes until you reach an oatmeal consistency. Remove the lemon peel and cinnamon stick and pour the cooked sweet rice into a serving dish; a shallow pie dish is ideal. Cool on the countertop for 20 minutes. Once the dish has cooled, move the dish to the fridge uncovered to cool completely, about 2–4 hours.

Once completely cooled, top with additional ground cinnamon in a cross pattern or just simply sprinkled on top.

FEEDING THE FRASERS

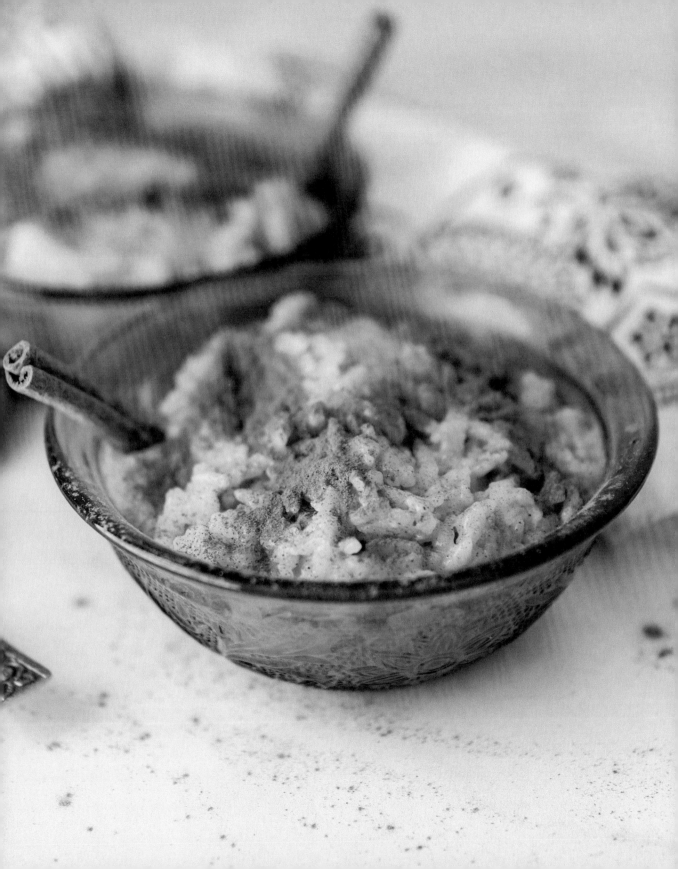

STRAWBERRY KIWI PIZZA

SERVES: *12*

PREP TIME: *30 MINUTES*

COOK TIME: *18 MINUTES*

COOKIE CRUST

1 cup (2 sticks) cold salted butter, cubed

2 ounces cold cream cheese, cubed

1 cup plus 2 tablespoons granulated sugar

¼ cup light brown sugar

1 egg

2 teaspoons vanilla extract

3 cups all-purpose flour

1 teaspoon baking powder

½ teaspoon salt

FROSTING

6 ounces cream cheese, room temperature

4 tablespoons salted butter, room temperature

½ cup honey

1 teaspoon vanilla extract

TOPPINGS

½ cup strawberries, sliced

2 kiwi, peeled and sliced

2 teaspoons fresh mint, sliced thin

MY MOM sold kitchen gadgets for a very popular brand in the mid-1990s. She'd host parties for friends and family, making various dishes with the kitchen tools to show their use. I'd assist in the kitchen and play hostess, filling up the guests' glasses of wine and passing around trays of samples. This recipe is a re-creation of one of those passed samples. For a good part of my childhood, it was what I requested on my birthday instead of a birthday cake. My love for cream cheese started at a young age.

Place the cold butter, cream cheese, granulated sugar, brown sugar, egg, and vanilla in the bowl of a food processor. Pulse 12–15 times to combine the ingredients. Add the flour, baking powder, and salt. Pulse an additional 10 times until the dough forms.

Press the cookie dough into a parchment-lined quarter baking sheet. Chill the dough in the freezer for 10 minutes while the oven preheats.

Preheat the oven to 350°F/177°C.

Bake for 15–18 minutes or until it's lightly browned. Remove from the oven. Cool for 5 minutes in the baking sheet before transferring the sugar cookie crust to a wire rack to complete cooling, about 30 minutes.

While the crust cools, prepare the frosting. In a medium bowl, beat the cream cheese, butter, honey, and vanilla using a hand mixer until smooth.

Once the crust is completely cooled, spread the frosting out evenly. Top with sliced strawberries and kiwi. Sprinkle with mint and cut into 12 even squares for serving.

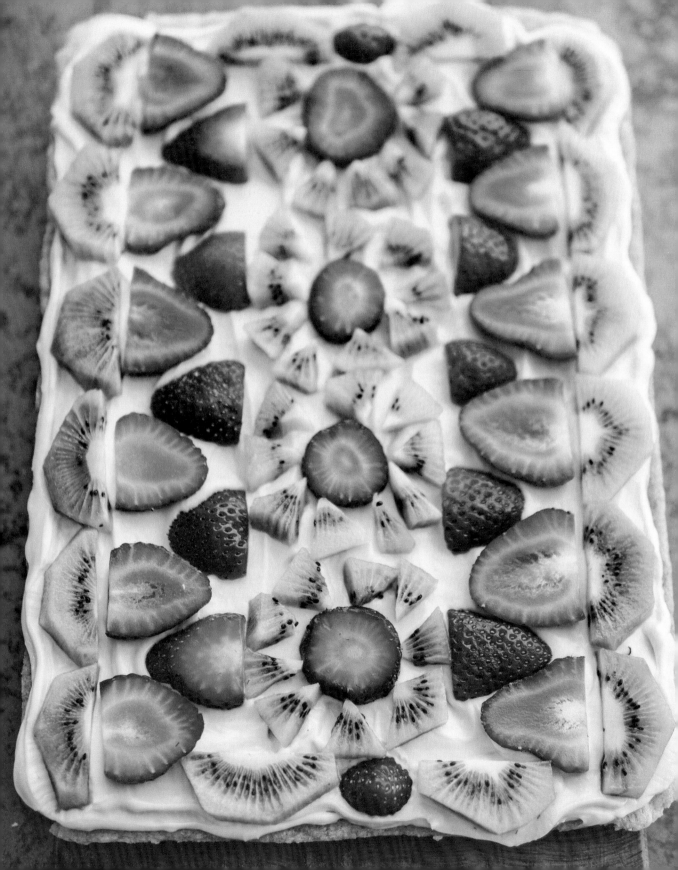

MINI STONE FRUIT TARTS

YIELDS: 12 TARTS
PREP TIME: 10 MINUTES
COOK TIME: 18–20 MINUTES

1 package puff pastry sheets, thawed

8 ounces Honey-Walnut Whipped Cream Cheese (see page 48 for recipe)

¼ cup coarse sugar for sprinkling (coconut sugar or sugar in the raw)

3 stone fruit, sliced (nectarines, peaches, plums, apricots)

1 egg whisked

1 tablespoon honey

THIS IS a simple dessert that's not too sweet and uses up some leftovers. What's better than that? If you've whipped up a batch of the Honey-Walnut Whipped Cream Cheese for your breakfast bagels and now have a craving for dessert after dinner, bust it out and either use up what you have left, or portion it out so you still have enough for your bagel the next morning. I love being able to repurpose things in my fridge and feel like I'm really making the most of mealtime.

Preheat the oven to 425°F/220°C. Line two baking sheets with parchment paper and set aside.

On a lightly floured surface using a lightly floured rolling pin, roll the pastry sheets out in each direction until about ⅛-inch thick rectangle. Cut into 12 4×3-inch rectangles. Lay each rectangle onto the prepared baking sheets.

To the center of each rectangle, smear 1–2 tablespoons of Honey-Walnut Whipped Cream Cheese. Sprinkle the centers with a pinch or two of the coarse sugar. Place 3–4 slices of stone fruit into the cream cheese. Curl up the edges of the puff pastry to touch the fruit. Brush the edges with egg wash and sprinkle the tops with an additional 1–2 teaspoons of coarse sugar.

Bake in the oven for 18–20 minutes or until the puff pastry is golden and the fruit is tender. Remove from the oven, cool on the baking sheet for 2 minutes before moving to a wire rack to cool slightly before serving. Drizzle with honey and serve while warm (not hot!).

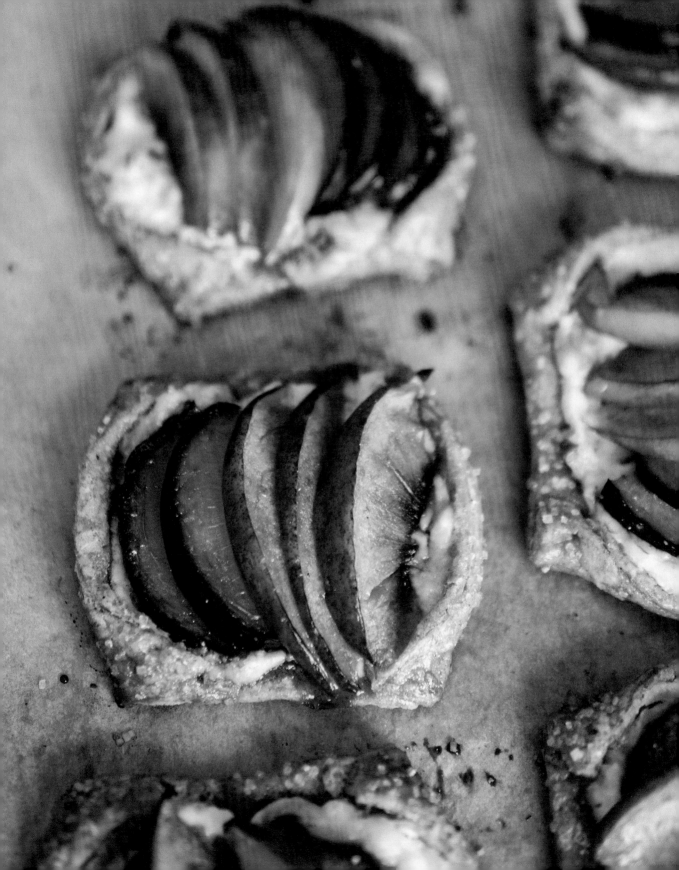

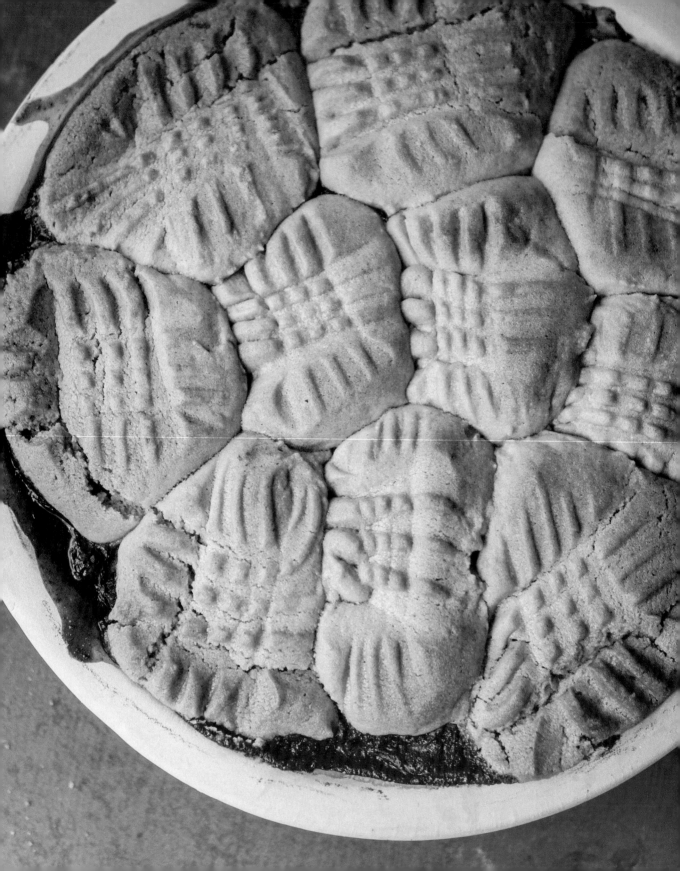

GOOEY PEANUT BUTTER & JELLY PIE

SERVES: 8

PREP TIME: 25 MINUTES

COOK TIME: 50 MINUTES

4 cups frozen mixed berries

½ cup plus 2 tablespoons granulated sugar, divided

1 tablespoon cornstarch

1 teaspoon lemon juice

¼ teaspoon vanilla extract

1⅓ cup all-purpose flour

½ teaspoon baking soda

¼ teaspoon baking powder

¼ teaspoon kosher salt

½ cup (1 stick) butter, softened

½ cup packed brown sugar

1 large egg, room temperature

¾ cup creamy peanut butter

GET READY for nostalgia to take over with every bite of this dessert. The cookie topping crisps on the outside and stays gooey on the inside, giving you the swirl of PB&J with every bite. Skip the brown paper bag lunches and dive headfirst into the dessert course.

Preheat the oven to 350°F/177°C.

In a lightly greased large pie dish, toss the frozen berries, 2 tablespoons of granulated sugar, cornstarch, lemon juice, and vanilla extract. Bake for 20 minutes.

While the berries are baking, prepare the cookie topping. In a medium bowl, stir the flour, baking soda, baking powder, and salt. Set aside. In a separate large bowl, beat the butter using a hand mixer until pale and fluffy, about 2 minutes. Add the ½ cup of granulated sugar and brown sugar, beat for an additional 1 minute until smooth. Add the egg and peanut butter and mix well until combined.

Add the dry ingredients into the bowl and mix with a silicone spatula until the cookie dough is smooth. Scoop the dough into 10–12 large balls and roll into a smooth ball between your palms; dampen your hands slightly if the dough begins to stick. Place the cookie balls on a sheet of parchment paper, and use a long pronged fork to flatten and create a crisscross pattern.

Remove the berries from the oven, place the cookies on top of the berries, and return the dish to the oven for 25–30 minutes. Remove from the oven and allow to cool for 5–10 minutes to set before serving. Serve warm and topped with a scoop of vanilla ice cream.

PRETZEL, HAZELNUT & PEANUT BUTTER ICEBOX CAKE

YIELDS: 12 CUPS

PREP TIME: 15 MINUTES (PLUS 3 HOURS CHILLING)

COOK TIME: 0 MINUTES

2⅔ cups heavy whipping cream, divided

1 (15-ounce) can sweetened condensed milk

½ cup creamy peanut butter

36 honey graham cracker squares

1 cup roasted hazelnuts, roughly chopped and divided

1 cup semisweet chocolate chips

1 cup pretzel sticks, lightly crushed

THE TITLE says it all. Combining all the best flavors and ingredients into one bite, and on top of it, it tastes like an ice cream cake without having to make ice cream. Are you sold? If you need more convincing, it comes together quickly, and it pairs great with a backyard BBQ in the summer.

Line a square 8x8 baking dish with parchment paper; be sure the paper hangs over the edges slightly for easy lifting when ready to slice and serve. Set aside.

Pour 2 cups of heavy whipping cream into the bowl of a stand mixer. Using the whisk attachment, set the mixer to high and beat the cream for 3–4 minutes until light and fluffy. Add the sweetened condensed milk and creamy peanut butter. Whisk for an additional 1 minute until fully incorporated and fluffy.

Create the base layer of the cake by placing graham cracker squares in the bottom of the parchment-lined dish. Cover the crackers with ⅓ of the peanut butter whipped cream. Add another layer of crackers and peanut butter whipped cream. Add a handful of chopped hazelnuts to the middle layer of peanut butter whipped cream. Repeat this process until you've completed 3 layers of peanut butter whipped cream, and close the top of the cake with another layer of crackers. Chill the icebox cake in the freezer for 2 hours.

After two hours, remove the cake from the freezer. In a microwave-safe bowl, heat ⅔ cup of heavy whipping cream in 20-second intervals until hot, about 1½ minutes total. Add the semisweet chocolate chips and allow them to sit in the hot cream for 1 minute. Begin to mix the chocolate and cream until the chocolate chips are

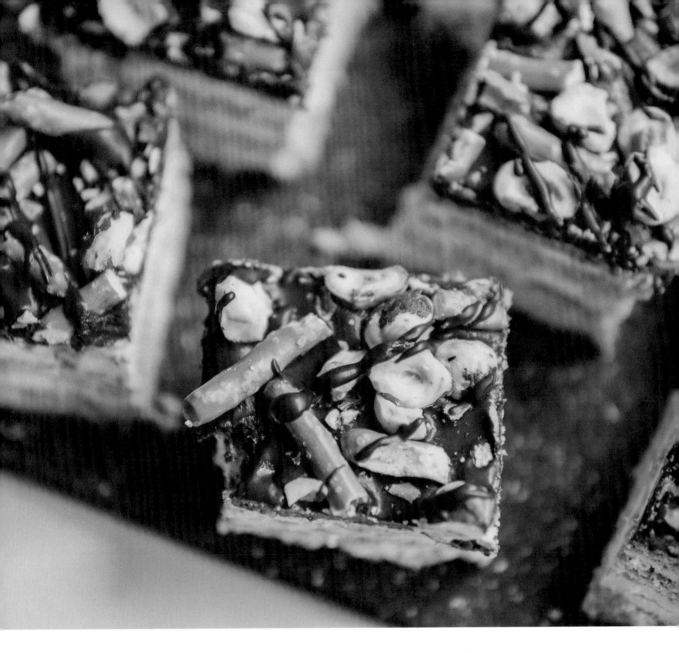

fully melted and the mixture is smooth. Pour the chocolate mixture on top of the cake, reserving 2–3 tablespoons of chocolate to drizzle on top. Evenly distribute the remaining hazelnuts and the lightly crushed pretzels. Drizzle the toppings with the remaining chocolate. Freeze for 1 hour.

Remove the cake from the freezer and rest on the counter for 10–15 minutes before slicing.

CARROT CAKE CHEESECAKE

SERVES: 4
PREP TIME: 20 MINUTES
COOK TIME: 100 MINUTES

CARROT CAKE

2½ cups all-purpose flour

2 teaspoons baking powder

1 teaspoon baking soda

½ teaspoon salt

1½ teaspoons ground cinnamon

1 teaspoon ground ginger

¼ teaspoon ground nutmeg

¼ teaspoon ground cloves

4 large eggs

1½ cups packed dark brown sugar

½ cup granulated sugar

1 teaspoon vanilla extract

1 cup high-quality olive oil

2 cups grated carrots

1 cup golden raisins

2 cups toasted pecans, chopped and divided

CHEESECAKE FILLING

16 ounces cream cheese, room temperature

⅓ cup sour cream

⅔ cup white sugar

2 eggs

2 teaspoons vanilla extract

THE LOVE child of two household favorites, the classic cheesecake and carrot cake. For every special occasion, I had to choose which family favorite to create. Now, we've got a one-stop shop bringing the best of both worlds together in one cake pan. We ate a lot of this cake in the summer of 2020. Many rounds of testing to get the cake just right! This cake is a labor of love and a marathon, not a sprint. It's all about that winning bite at the finish line!

Preheat the oven to 350°F/177°C. Place a roasting pan on the bottom rack of the oven filled with water to create moisture in the oven.

Prepare a springform pan by spraying the inside with cooking spray and lightly flouring. Stand the pan up and tap all sides to make sure the flour lightly coats all areas, then discard excess flour. Cut a piece of parchment paper to line the bottom of the pan. Set aside.

To make the cake portion, whisk the flour, baking powder, baking soda, salt, cinnamon, ginger, nutmeg, and cloves until combined in a medium bowl. In a separate large bowl, whisk the eggs, brown sugar, granulated sugar, vanilla, and oil until combined. Pour the dry ingredients into the wet ingredients and gently fold until combined. Next, fold in the carrots, raisins, and ½ cup of pecans. Be careful not to overmix. Pour the batter into a prepared springform pan and set aside to prepare the cheesecake filling.

In the bowl of a stand mixer, add the cream cheese, sour cream, and sugar. Whip until fluffy, about 3 minutes. Add the eggs one at a time. Whip until smooth. Add the vanilla and whip an additional 30 seconds. Pour the cheesecake filling over the cake layer.

CREAM CHEESE FROSTING

8 ounces cream cheese, room temperature

¼ cup unsalted butter, room temperature

2 cups powdered sugar

1–1½ tablespoons heavy cream

½ teaspoon vanilla extract

Pinch salt

Using a large piece of aluminum foil, create a tent over the cake pan, securing loosely on two sides of the cake. Place the cake in the center of the oven and close the door.

Bake for 70–80 minutes until the cheesecake is set with a slight jiggle in the middle. After 40 minutes, check the roasting pan and quickly refill with water as needed. At the 70–80 minute mark, remove the aluminum foil and bake for an additional 10 minutes. Turn off the oven, crack the door to the oven, and leave the cheesecake inside for an additional 30 minutes. After 30 minutes, remove the cheesecake from the oven and place the pan on a wire cooling rack to completely cool, about 2 hours. Once completely cooled, cover and refrigerate 8 hours or overnight.

To make the frosting, beat the cream cheese and butter in a large bowl with a handheld mixer on medium until smooth. Add the powdered sugar, cream, and vanilla and whip until just combined. Taste the frosting and add a pinch of salt as needed.

To decorate the chilled cheesecake, remove the springform pan and place on a serving plate. Top the cake with the cream cheese frosting and the remaining 1½ cups of toasted pecans.

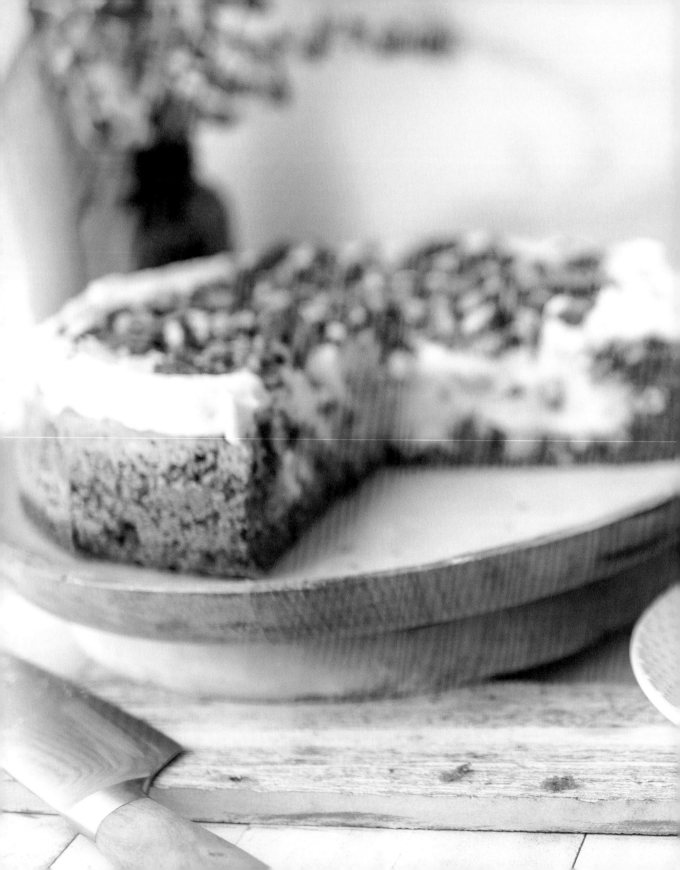

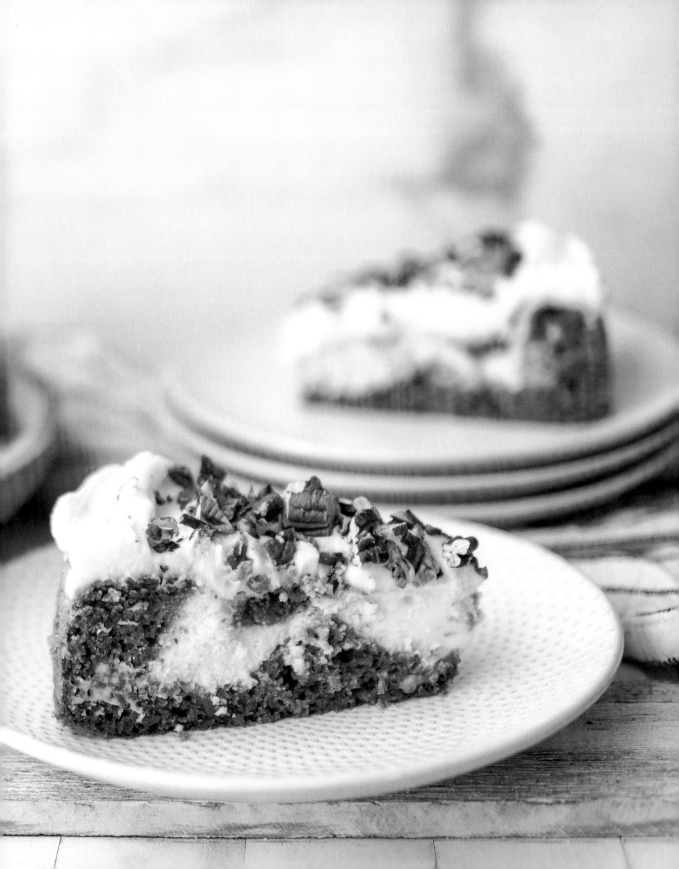

CAMPFIRE COOKIES

YIELDS: 12 LARGE
COOKIES
PREP TIME: 15 MINUTES
COOK TIME: 12 MINUTES

YIELDS: *12 LARGE
COOKIES*
PREP TIME: *15 MINUTES*
COOK TIME: *12 MINUTES*

1¾ cups all-purpose flour

1 cup cocoa powder

2 teaspoons baking soda

½ teaspoon salt

1 teaspoon cinnamon

1 teaspoon espresso powder

1 cup salted butter, room temperature

1 cup granulated sugar

¾ cup brown sugar

2 eggs, room temperature

1 tablespoon vanilla extract

1½ cups chocolate chips

1 sleeve graham crackers

40–60 mini marshmallows

Flaky salt for sprinkling

IF I'M remembering correctly, this recipe came about after the countless stare-downs with the box of graham crackers in my pantry. Every time I opened the pantry door, there it was begging to be put to good use. While I didn't step too far from s'mores, I was happy to give this pantry item a new life. You can make 24 small cookies or 12 large cookies with this batter. For large cookies, follow the directions below for about 12 minutes of baking time. For small cookies, adjust to 8–10 minutes total baking time.

Preheat the oven to 375°F/190°C.

In a large mixing bowl, sift the flour, cocoa powder, baking soda, salt, cinnamon, and espresso powder. Set aside.

In a separate large bowl, cream the butter using a hand mixer for about 1 minute until fluffy and pale. Add the granulated sugar and brown sugar. Beat for 1 minute until well combined. Add eggs and vanilla, this time mixing until just combined.

Into the bowl of butter and sugar, add the dry ingredients, folding with a wooden spoon or silicone spatula until fully incorporated. Stir in the chocolate chips.

Place the sleeve of graham crackers into a food processor, pulse into a fine crumb. Pour the contents into a shallow dish and set aside.

Using a ¼ cup scoop or measuring cup, scoop the cookie batter. Using your hands, roll the batter into a ball. Roll the ball into the dish of graham cracker crumbs to coat. Place each rolled cookie onto a parchment-lined baking sheet. Use the bottom of the measuring cup to slightly flatten.

Bake the cookies for 8 minutes. The cookies should begin to crack on top. Remove from the oven. Gently push

FEEDING THE FRASERS

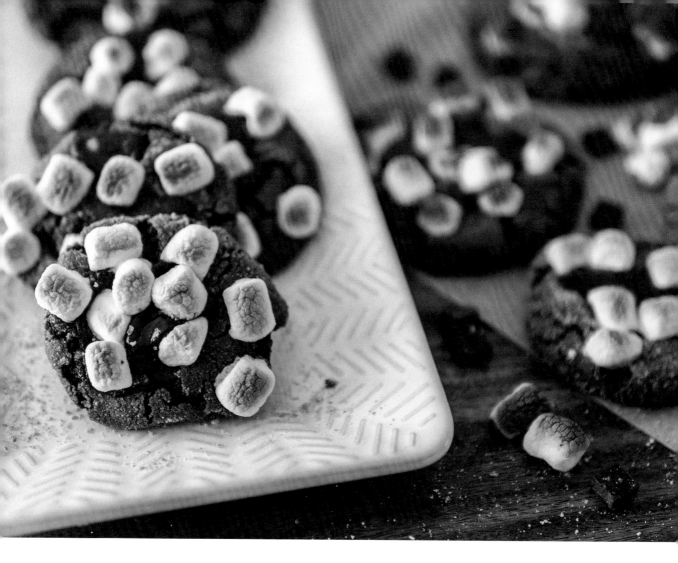

a small handful of mini marshmallows into the top of each cookie and sprinkle with a pinch of flaky salt. Return to the oven for an additional 4 minutes.

Cool on the baking sheet for 5 minutes to set. Carefully move each cookie to a wire cooling rack to cool completely.

PRO TIP

Be sure to space the cookies out, as they will spread as they bake. On a full baking sheet, I'll typically do 8 cookies to allow enough space. It's worth working in batches to ensure a perfect bake.

ANZAC BISCUITS

YIELDS: 2 DOZEN BISCUITS
PREP TIME: 10 MINUTES
COOK TIME: 13–15 MINUTES

1 cup all-purpose flour

1 cup rolled oats

¾ cup shredded coconut

⅛ teaspoon salt

¼ cup granulated sugar

¼ cup brown sugar

1 teaspoon orange zest

½ cup butter, melted

2 tablespoons golden syrup (or honey)

1½ teaspoons baking soda

2 tablespoons boiling water

WE WERE lucky enough to have some Australian friends, and thankfully, they also like to EAT. This is not your typical American cookie. It's rooted in Australian history as the biscuits sent off to the soldiers during World War I because the ingredients in the biscuit wouldn't spoil in transport. Our Aussie friends have taste tested many of the recipes in this book between training sessions at the gym; it's only right to include an Australian treat since they are very much a part of our well-fed family.

Preheat the oven to 350°F/175°C. Line two baking sheets with parchment paper and set aside.

In a medium bowl, stir the flour, oats, coconut, salt, granulated sugar, brown sugar, and orange zest until well combined.

In a separate medium bowl, melt the butter in the microwave in 15- to 30-second intervals. Add the golden syrup (or honey) to the hot butter and stir until well combined.

In a small bowl, stir the baking soda and boiling water until dissolved. Add the baking soda mixture to the butter and golden syrup. Be cautious, as it will react and bubble as it hits the butter mixture. Stir to combine.

Make a well in the oats mixture, pour the wet ingredients into the well, and stir until the biscuit batter is combined and no dry bits remain.

Using a tablespoon scoop or measuring spoon, scoop 24 cookies. Roll each cookie slightly between your palms and place on a cookie sheet. (I baked these in 3 batches with 8 cookies per sheet to allow enough room for the cookies to spread.) Slightly flatten the

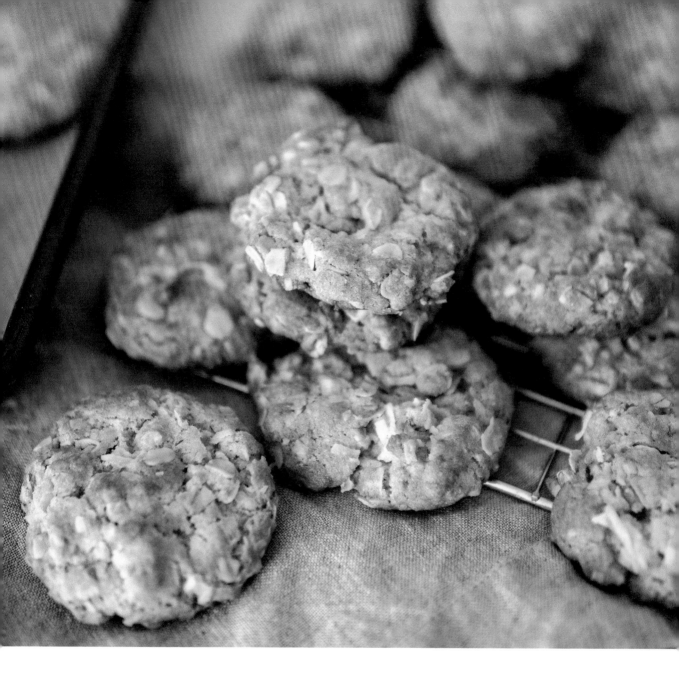

cookies with your fingers or the back of your scoop. Bake for 10–12 minutes until golden brown.

Remove the cookies from the oven, place on a wire rack to cool on the baking sheet for 3 minutes. Remove the cookies from the baking sheet and place directly on the cooling rack to finish cooling.

SALTED BROWN BUTTER CHOCOLATE CHIP COOKIES

YIELDS: 4–6 COOKIES

PREP TIME: 40 MINUTES

COOK TIME: 25 MINUTES

8 tablespoons salted butter, browned and slightly cooled

½ cup light brown sugar, packed

⅓ cup granulated sugar

1 egg

1 egg yolk

½ tablespoon pure vanilla extract

2 teaspoons cornstarch

1 teaspoon baking soda

¾ teaspoon sea salt

1¾ cups all-purpose flour

½ cup mini chocolate morsels

½ cup mega chocolate chunks

1–2 tablespoons flaky sea salt

EVER WALK into a hip coffee shop or a classic bakery and drool at the baked goods in the display case? At this amazing coffee shop in Columbus, Ohio, the selection of biscuits and jam, cinnamon rolls, and danishes are enough to satisfy. What caught my eye was the giant chocolate chip cookie. It was as if they rolled four cookies into one. Genius! Who decided 1- or 2-ounce cookie scoops were the standard? What if I want a 4- or 6-ounce cookie that I need both hands to hold? That's what I've given you here, the freedom to choose your cookie size!

In a large bowl, whisk the browned butter with brown sugar and granulated sugar until well combined. Add the egg, egg yolk, and vanilla, whisk to combine.

In a separate bowl, whisk the cornstarch, baking soda, sea salt, and all-purpose flour. Add the dry ingredients to the bowl of wet ingredients. Use a wooden spoon to incorporate. Lastly, add the mini chocolate morsels and mega chocolate chunks to the cookie batter. Mix until just combined.

Using a food scale, divide the batter into 6 (4-ounce) portions. Roll the dough into a ball, place on a parchment-lined baking sheet, and freeze for at least 30 minutes (ideally 1 hour since these are *big* cookies). When ready to bake, preheat the oven 325°F/162°C.

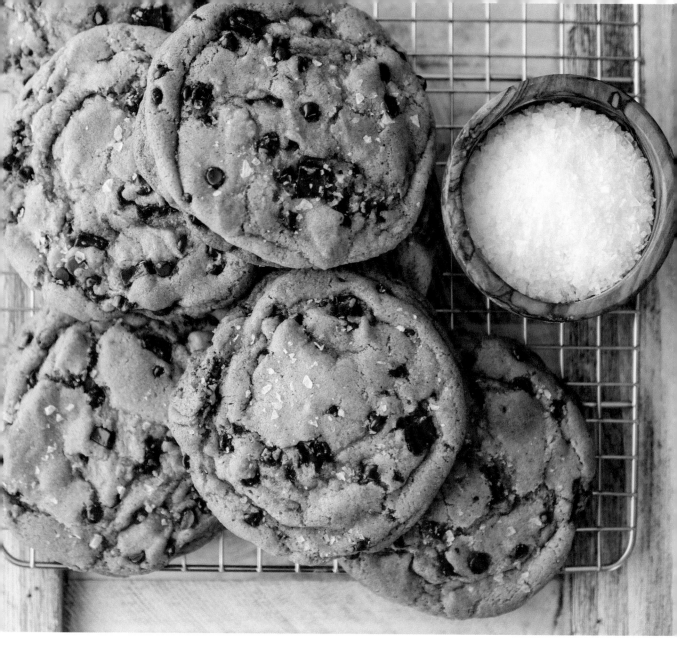

Remove the cookies from the freezer and place directly into the heated oven. Bake for 22–25 minutes or until desired doneness (we like them slightly underbaked). When the cookies are done, remove them from the oven and sprinkle with flaky sea salt. Allow the cookies to cool on the baking sheet for 5 minutes to set before moving to a wire rack to cool.

WINTER CITRUS OLIVE OIL CAKE

SERVES: 10–12
PREP TIME: 15 MINUTES
COOK TIME: 40–45 MINUTES

CAKE

2 tablespoons grapefruit zest

1 cup granulated sugar

2 large eggs

½ cup grapefruit juice

¾ cup olive oil

1½ cups all-purpose flour

½ teaspoon baking powder

¼ teaspoon baking soda

¼ teaspoon salt

FROSTING

6 tablespoons olive oil

¾ cup powdered sugar

Pinch kosher salt

TOPPINGS

1 grapefruit, cut into segments for serving

1 tablespoon mint, finely minced

¼ cup roasted pistachios, crushed or finely diced

THIS WAS the first recipe I wrote for this book. I had just come home from an olive harvest in California at an olive grove, where I tasted fresh EVOO from the trees. The olive oil, picked at peak freshness and pressed on-site, is bright in color and grassy in flavor with a little natural spice on the back of your tongue. I had no idea how delicious a single pantry ingredient could be. I want to highlight the ingredient in a new way and give my well-fed followers an experience with olive oil like I'd had.

Preheat the oven to 350°F/177°C. To prepare a springform pan (or regular 8-inch cake pan) spray the pan with cooking spray and add a small scoop of flour. Turn and tap to run the flour over every inch of the pan surface. Tap out any excess flour over the trash bin or sink. Cut a piece of parchment paper to line the bottom of the pan for easy lift out of the pan once the cake is baked and cooled. Set the prepared pan aside.

In a large bowl, work the grapefruit zest and sugar with your hands until fragrant. To the bowl, add the eggs, grapefruit juice, and olive oil. Beat using a hand mixer on medium-high speed for 2 minutes until bubbly.

In a separate bowl, sift the flour, baking powder, baking soda, and salt.

Add the dry ingredients into the wet. Gently fold until no dry bits of flour remain. Pour the batter into the center of a prepared springform or 8-inch cake pan. Bake the cake for 40-45 minutes or until a toothpick dipped into the center of the cake comes out clean.

While the cake bakes, prepare the frosting and garnishes. In a medium bowl, whisk the olive oil, powdered sugar, and kosher salt and set aside. In

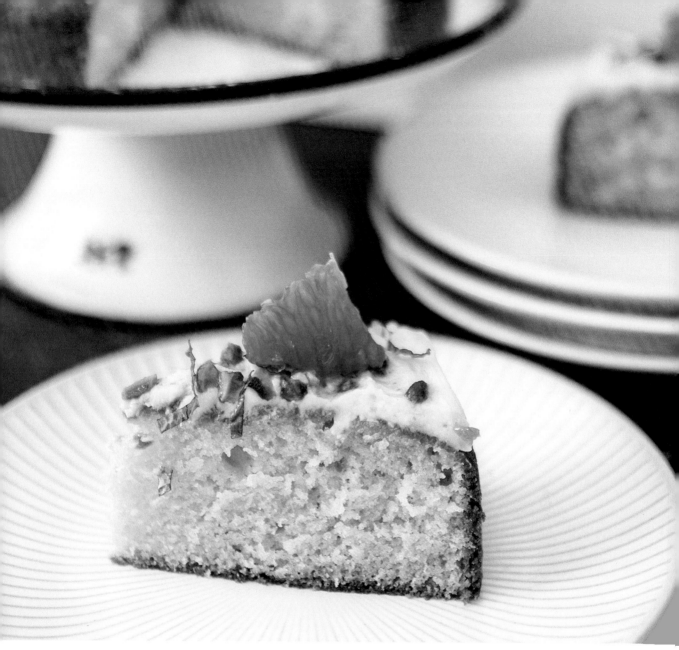

another bowl, toss the grapefruit segments with the mint, cover and refrigerate until ready to serve.

Remove cake from the oven and cool in the pan for 30 minutes. At 30 minutes, remove the sides of the springform pan and cool for an additional 30 minutes. Once completely cooled, flip onto a plate to remove the bottom pan and parchment paper and flip again onto a serving dish or cake stand.

Frost the cake, sprinkle with crushed pistachios, and top with slices of fresh grapefruit.

DIABLO BROWNIES

SERVES: 12

PREP TIME: 10 MINUTES

COOK TIME: 30 MINUTES

½ cup all-purpose flour

½ cup unsweetened cocoa powder

1 teaspoon baking powder

½ teaspoon cayenne pepper

1 teaspoon cinnamon

¾ teaspoon ground ginger

1 cup salted butter

2 cups semisweet chocolate chips

1 cup granulated sugar

½ cup brown sugar

1 tablespoon vanilla extract

2 teaspoons espresso powder (or instant coffee granules)

4 large eggs, at room temperature

1 teaspoon flaky salt

BROWNIES ARE my kryptonite. I don't make them often, truthfully, hardly ever. I cannot control myself around a tray of fudgy brownies. Not to mention these Diablo Brownies. The combination of kicking flavors and fudgy squares is an irresistible combination for me.

Preheat the oven to 375°F/190°C.

In a large bowl, sift the flour, cocoa powder, baking powder, cayenne pepper, cinnamon, and ginger. Set aside.

In a separate large bowl, microwave the butter and 1½ cups of chocolate chips (stir at 30-second intervals) until melted and smooth. Stir in the sugars, vanilla, and espresso powder.

In a small bowl, whisk the eggs for 1 minute until bubbly on top. Stir the eggs into the melted chocolate mix. Add the dry ingredients to the melted chocolate mix. Stir until just combined. Lastly, stir in the remaining ½ cup of chocolate chips.

Evenly spread the batter into a parchment-lined square 8x8 baking dish. Bake for 28–30 minutes or until the brownies are just set. Remove from the oven, sprinkle with flaky salt, and let cool for at least 5 minutes before slicing.

SNACKS & SWEETS

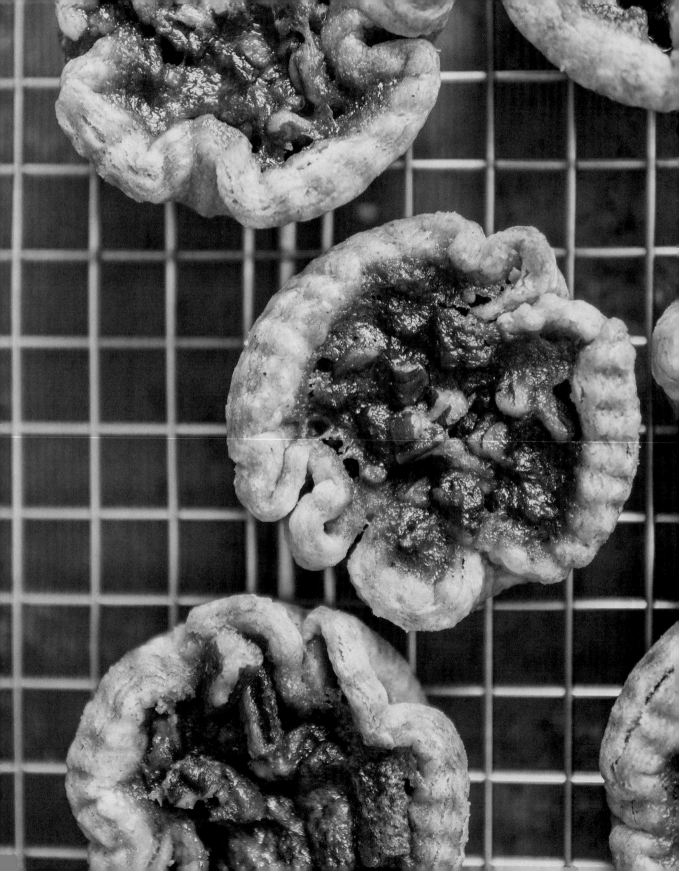

BUTTER TARTS

SERVES: 16
PREP TIME: 75 MINUTES
COOK TIME: 11–13 MINUTES

DOUGH

2 cups all-purpose flour

½ cup whole-wheat flour

1 teaspoon ground cinnamon

½ teaspoon salt

1 cup cold salted butter, cubed

½ cup ice-cold water

FILLING

¼ cup salted butter, room temperature

⅔ cup brown sugar

¼ teaspoon salt

2 tablespoons golden syrup (or light corn syrup)

1 teaspoon vanilla extract

2 large eggs

¾ cup pecan pieces

THESE GOOEY tarts are a famous Canadian treat. Every summer, after the CrossFit Games, we'd retreat to a family camp in Ontario, Canada, for a week or two on the lake. Pure vacation. The days consist of waking up, grabbing a cup of coffee, and heading down to the dock. We'd sit on that dock for hours staring at the lake, listening to the loons, and chatting about the year and our future until our bellies growled. A quick walk up to the cabin and a tray of butter tarts would always be waiting to satisfy the hunger. Meals weren't exactly balanced, but that's why it's called vacation—you let go of balance and just give in to enjoying!

To make the dough, mix the all-purpose flour, whole-wheat flour, cinnamon, and salt. Add the cubes of butter. Working quickly with your hands, toss the butter with the flour to coat. Pinch the cubes between your fingers and recoat with the flour. When all the cubes have been flattened and distributed, add the ice-cold water and mix with your hands until the dough is shaggy. Turn the dough out onto a lightly floured surface. Fold, press, and fold the dough again until it forms a smooth disc. Wrap the disc tightly in cling wrap and chill in the fridge for 30 minutes.

Once the dough has chilled and rested, roll it out on a lightly floured surface until it's about a ¼-inch thick. Using a large biscuit cutter, punch out 16 cuts of dough. Lightly flour the surface as needed and roll each cut out slightly. Once all the dough is rolled out, gently press the dough into a well-greased muffin tin. Each circle of dough should sit into the muffin tin and crawl up the sides to create a cup for the filling. Place the dough-filled muffin tin in the freezer for 20 minutes while you prepare the filling and preheat the oven.

Preheat the oven to 450°F/230°C.

In a medium bowl, beat the softened butter using a hand mixer. Add the brown sugar and salt, beat until smooth, about 2 minutes. Add the golden syrup, vanilla extract, and eggs and mix until combined. Lastly, add the pecans and fold with a silicone spatula.

Fill each cup ⅔ of the way with the filling. Bake for 11–13 minutes. Cool in the muffin tin for 10 minutes, carefully remove each tart from the pan, and continue cooling on a wire rack for an additional 10–15 minutes to set the filling.

AFTERWORD

What an adventure it was writing, cooking, and photographing this book! There were days of immediate success, the recipes that hit on the first try after scribbling down the idea. Then there were days of remake after remake to get it just right. I'm pretty sure I made and tested the Carrot Cake Cheesecake nine times. Yes, nine times. I am forever grateful for this opportunity to learn. To create. To make and remake! I started this cooking journey to learn how to cook, and this book has taught me so much more than just the perfect recipe for Sausage Buttermilk Biscuits, Zesty Orange Salmon Poké Bowls, and Diablo Brownies. Thank you for showing up, for being courageous in your kitchen, and for sharing your creations with friends and family.

INDEX

INDEX